# Muscular Dystrophy

Raymond A. Huml
Editor

# Muscular Dystrophy

A Concise Guide

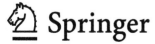 Springer

*Editor*
Raymond A. Huml
Biosimilars Center of Excellence
Quintiles Inc.
Durham, NC, USA

ISBN 978-3-319-17361-0        ISBN 978-3-319-17362-7    (eBook)
DOI 10.1007/978-3-319-17362-7

Library of Congress Control Number: 2015939175

Springer Cham Heidelberg New York Dordrecht London

Printed on acid-free paper

Springer International Publishing AG Switzerland is part of Springer Science+Business Media (www.springer.com)

# Foreword

The various forms of muscular dystrophy (MD) are rare diseases, but ones that create enormous consequences for both patients and their caregivers. Since the typical age of onset falls within childhood, patients' primary caregivers are usually their parents. Once their child has been diagnosed with MD, these parents must face a new set of demands on their time, energy, emotions, and finances, usually all at a time when they are also hard at work dealing with the day-to-day demands of their jobs and careers. In a very real sense, MD affects many more individuals than those who are diagnosed as patients. This group of diseases truly deserves our attention.

The term MD refers to many diseases, differing in age-of-onset of clinical symptoms, degree of severity, and underlying genetic causes. Nonetheless, all share the key similarity of progressive muscular weakening, resulting in loss of mobility, agility, and bodily movement. While the upper arms and upper legs often display such weakness first, multiple other organs can be affected, including the diaphragm and chest muscles, stomach, intestines, brain, and even heart. Quality of life, therefore, can be severely affected.

We are now aware that each type of MD results from a different specific genetic defect affecting the proteins governing muscular function and integrity. Genetic programming underlying muscular function is enormously complex, and each form of MD originates from different genetic mutations. For example, the Duchenne and Becker forms of MD are caused by different mutations in the gene for dystrophin, a protein very important for maintaining normal muscle structure and function. Loss of dystrophin functionality causes muscle fragility, leading to progressive weakness and loss of ambulatory ability, usually during childhood and teenage years. Heterogeneity of disease origins creates difficulties in determining how best to approach the development of pharmaceutical therapies, since successful treatment of each of the various types of MD which can be expected to require a different drug to reach and interact with each specific target receptor. Fortunately, advances are finally being achieved in this regard, along with many other important facets of addressing this disease group, as detailed in this book.

I first met Raymond A. Huml, this book's Editor, who also authored and coauthored several of its chapters, when we were working together at Quintiles, a large, global Contract Research Organization (CRO) that assists pharmaceutical, biotechnology, and medical device companies around the world to bring important new products to market successfully. During his ongoing career in the pharmaceutical industry, Dr. Huml has gained tremendous experience in numerous aspects of bringing new drugs to market. To name but a few, these include how to perform due diligence in choosing the best pharmaceutical investments (subject of yet another book he authored), becoming an expert in the worldwide regulatory landscapes with which development of new drugs must comply, and becoming a major U.S. expert in the emerging area of organic "biosimilar" drug development.

These facts, however, are only one of the facets of what makes him the perfect person to assemble the distinguished group of authors who share their knowledge and insights in the following chapters. Dr. Huml is also a well-respected North Carolina veterinarian, who compassionately treated animal patients for many years and who currently sits on the Board of Visitors for North Carolina State University. Perhaps most pertinent of all, though is the fact that Ray and his wife Leslie are the parents of two children, both of whom suffer from MD: Meredith, who was diagnosed in 2003, and Jonathan, diagnosed in 2013, both suffer from facioscapulohumeral MD (FSHD). As the name reflects, the typical locations of the muscular weakening in FSHD are the face, shoulder girdle, and upper arms.

Thus, both Dr. Huml's personal experience and his professional expertise have provided him with a broad spectrum of insights regarding MD, from individual patient management, through the best currently available treatment options, all the way up to public health issues. At the individual patient level, he has learned, firsthand, the demands and challenges MD brings both to patients and their family members. At the treatment level, his successful global CRO career in pharmaceutical development provides him with the ability to identify and focus on the most potentially effective drugs, especially those currently under development. At the public health level, he is intimately familiar with the challenges along with numerous successful approaches to developing new drugs and then gaining regulatory approval for them. This propels them from laboratory benches to patient bedsides, resulting in large improvement in outcomes. He and his collaborators address these issues very well in this book.

The confluence of various recent occurrences makes this the perfect time for providing a concise but very inclusive reference and guide regarding MD. First, there remains a high unmet medical need for MD treatments. Second, increasing scientific knowledge about the root causes and disease mechanisms of various forms of MD is resulting in more focus on developing new, specific drug treatments. Third, awareness is now growing that MD patients were, all-too-often, left at the back of the line for the development of new medications. Patient advocacy groups, combined with public social media, are rapidly gaining influence. That, along with the solid foundation this book provides, should help voices in the MD therapeutic arena to be heard nationwide.

This concise guide to MD educates us on many levels and many topics, but always maintains its patient-centric focus: this humanity may be the book's greatest strength of all.

Ross M. Tonkens, MD
Science & Technology Accelerator Division
American Heart Association,
Morrisville, NC, USA

# Editor's Introduction

I was intimately introduced to muscular dystrophy (MD) when my daughter, Meredith, was diagnosed with FSHD at Duke University's Muscular Dystrophy Association (MDA) Center in 2003. My son, Jonathan, was diagnosed with the same affliction at the University of North Carolina at Chapel Hill in 2013.

Since the first diagnosis, I have reached out to multiple caregivers, hospitals, and organizations in an attempt to understand FSHD—the most common form of MD, although far from the best known—as well as to obtain stabilization options and understand the risks and benefits of potential treatments and surgical recommendations which required second, third, and fourth opinions. My personal experience with MD before my children's diagnoses was limited to information provided by Jerry Lewis and the MDA as they championed a treatment for Duchenne MD (DMD) over the last half a century.

The greatest help that my children and I have received has been via their direct caregivers. Some of these world-renowned caregivers have agreed to champion a greater awareness of MD by joining me as co-authors or individual authors for this book. This group of dedicated medical and scientific professionals includes physicians working on FSHD clinical trials, as well as experts directly working with patients, their families, and support organizations. In addition, the book benefits from a doctoral-level (candidate) physical therapist and orthotic expert. Our family has also greatly benefited from guidance provided from premier patient and family support organizations such as the FSH Society and the MDA.

This book uniquely benefits from authorship provided by Daniel P. Perez, cofounder of the FSH Society, who offers insights into MD as a person afflicted with FSHD. Daniel has personally testified before the U.S. Congress over a period spanning greater than two decades on behalf of patients afflicted with FSHD. Although no longer with us, I would like to note that Daniel's mother, Carol A. Perez, who was also afflicted with FSHD, was another founder of the FSH Society and up until almost the time of her passing, could be counted on to provide guidance and encouragement to those with FSHD or those caring for persons afflicted with FSHD. On this matter, I speak from personal experience.

This books also benefits from authorship provided by my daughter, Meredith L. Huml, who wrote Chapter 13. The chapter provides her patient's perspective, and that of a younger, nonscientist member of this book's authorship clan.

When my daughter was first diagnosed with FSHD, there were more gaps in our knowledge of FSHD inheritance and understanding of molecular targets was not advanced enough to warrant research investment by large pharmaceutical companies. The greatest clinical trial advances have been made over the last decade and, largely as a result of new targets, potential treatments are now garnering the clinical attention of big pharma and potential investors. For example, a recent review (December 4, 2014) of the Website *clinicaltrials.gov* yielded 138 clinical studies involving the treatment of DMD, 137 studies involving Becker MD (BMD), and 24 studies involving FSHD.

This is good news for patients afflicted with MD and their families because there has never been a time when more new treatments were being investigated at the laboratory bench or in the clinic. In addition, promising new laboratory animal models of MD—an important stepping stone in the drug development process—are being discovered and developed.

This book is mainly focused on the most prevalent type of MD, FSHD, and the most severe, DMD, and on BMD—which is mechanistically related to DMD. These three types of MD also appear to be garnering the most attention of the pharmaceutical industry in terms of research investment, and of the regulatory bodies that will need to approve future therapies, including the promulgation of global regulations. The book also mentions and highlights aspects of the other types of MD; however, they are not discussed in as much detail.

Many factors make this the right time for a concise book on MD. First, there exists a high unmet medical need for MD treatments. Second, breakthroughs in science, technology, and gene manipulation have elucidated, and are continuing to elucidate, new targets, and in 2014, tentative approval was granted in the EU for the first treatment for DMD. Indeed, in May 2014, advisors to European regulators (e.g., the Committee for Medicinal Products for Human Use or CHMP) recommended early tentative approval for PTC Therapeutics' (PTC) ataluren, a treatment for DMD to be marketed as Translarna™. If the European Commission grants conditional approval, this could be followed by full EU approval if the data from the ongoing Phase III trial are sufficiently compelling.

However, in parallel with all of this exploding science and early breakthroughs, there still exists a need for the patient, the family member, and the pharmaceutical executive to understand more about this rapidly changing landscape.

In essence, the pharmaceutical industry is continuing to look for ways to decrease risk while investing in products for the treatment of MD. With this increase in clinical pressure, international regulatory agencies, including the European Medicines Agency ( EMA), have responded, and are beginning to issue guidance to maximize the probability of technical success and registration for new MD products. In an unprecedented move, the FDA solicited draft guidance for industry in June 2014 from a DMD patient advocacy group, Parent Project Muscular Dystrophy or PPMD,[2] and my hope is that this milestone will encourage other advocacy groups advocating for patients with the other MDs and advocacy groups for patients with other rare diseases.

My sincere wish is that this guide can be used by families affected by MD, by persons afflicted with MD, by caregivers new to the MD space, by pharmaceutical executives studying potential treatments for MD, and by third party capital executives considering investment in MD treatments. We are at an exciting time and my hope is that we will see a fully approved product for DMD within the next year and a disease-modifying treatment of FSHD in either Europe or America before 2020.

# References

1. Garde D. PTC soars as EU changes its tune on the DMD-treating ataluren, FierceBiotech. 2014. http://www.fiercebiotech.com/story/ptc-soars-eu-changes-its-tune-dmd-treating-ataluren/2014-05-23. Accessed 7 Dec 2014.
2. First-ever patient-initiated "Guidance for Industry" for Duchenne muscular dystrophy submitted to FDA. PR Newswire. 2014. http://www.marketwatch.com/story/first-ever-patient-initiated-guidance-for-industry-for-duchenne-muscular-dystrophy-submitted-to-fda-2014-06-25. Accessed 5 Jul 2014.

# Acknowledgements

I wish to express my gratitude to Dr. Dennis Gillings, CBE, Chairman and Founder of Quintiles Transnational Corp, and World Dementia Envoy (as appointed by the UK Prime Minister to facilitate scientific and financial innovation related to the treatment of patients with dementia) especially for his personal support, but also for the opportunity to learn about the complex processes of pharmaceutical drug development and risk-based investing in pharmaceutical products over a 20+ year time frame; to Tom Pike, CEO of Quintiles, for his personal support of my publications and for providing me with the opportunity to serve in Quintiles Center for Integrated Drug Development; to Dr. Derek Winstanly, Chief Customer and Governance Officer and Executive Board Member, for his friendship, generous mentorship and insights into leadership; to Daniel P. Perez, President and Founder of the Facioscapulohumeral (FSH) Society for his friendship and unique clinical insights into the processes of MD; to Dr. Geoffrey Barker, former Chief Scientific and Medical Officer of Quintiles, for his generous mentorship, support of my family and historical coauthorship; for Dr. Ross Tonkens, for his generous mentorship, friendship, editorial support, and historical coauthorship; to my daughter and son, Meredith L. and Jonathan R. Huml, for their unique insights into patient advocacy; to Drs. Kathryn Wagner, Zheng (Jane) Fan, Robert K. Lark, Edward C. Smith, Jean K. Mah for their generous co-authorship as well as their astute clinical ability, encouragement, and support of my family; to Laura Case for her patience, support, and keen insights into physical therapy, orthotic and mobility devices; and to Drs. Rick Turner and Jill Dawson for their unwavering friendship and editorial assistance.

# Contents

# Contributors

**Laura E. Case, D.P.T., M.S., P.C.S., C./N.D.T.** Division of Physical Therapy, Department of Community and Family Medicine, Duke University Medical Center, Durham, NC, USA

**Zheng (Jane) Fan, M.D.** Department of Neurology, University of North Carolina at Chapel Hill, Chapel Hill, NC, USA

**Elizabeth W. Hubbard, M.D.** Department of Orthopedic Surgery, Duke University Medical Center, Lenox Baker Children's Hospital, Durham, NC, USA

**Meredith L. Huml** % Raymond A. Huml, Quintiles Inc., Durham, NC, USA

**Raymond A. Huml, M.S., D.V.M., R.A.C.** Biosimilars Center of Excellence, Quintiles Inc., Durham, NC, USA

**Robert K. Lark, M.D., M.S.** Department of Orthopedic Surgery, Duke University Medical Center, Lenox Baker Children's Hospital, Durham, NC, USA

**Jean K. Mah, M.D., M.Sc.** Department of Pediatrics and Clinical Neurosciences, University of Calgary, Alberta Children's Hospital, Calgary, AB, Canada

**Elba Yesi Gerena Maldonado, M.D.** Department of Rehabilitation Medicine, University of Washington, Seattle, WA, USA

**Daniel P. Perez** FSH Society, Inc., Lexington, MA, USA

**Kathryn R. Wagner, M.D., Ph.D.** Kennedy Krieger Institute, Center for Genetic Muscle Disorders, Baltimore, MD, USA

# About the Editor

**Raymond A. Huml, M.S., D.V.M., R.A.C.** is Executive Director, Strategic Drug Development, and Head, Global Biosimilars Strategic Planning, at Quintiles, Inc. Dr. Huml has written over 50 articles and 2 books on a variety of clinical and pharmaceutical topics, including authoring MD articles and editing and co-authoring this book for *Springer* Publishing. He is also a member and supporter of the FSH Society.

Dr. Huml was previously Head of Global Due Diligence in Corporate Development for Quintiles Inc. He has more than 25 years of experience in the biopharmaceutical industry, working on all major investment transactions while at Quintiles, involving almost $3.0 billion in capital on alliances with biotechnology and pharmaceutical partners of all sizes. Earlier in his career, Dr. Huml worked in biostatistics, medical writing, and regulatory affairs in Quintiles' clinical development services group. Dr. Huml holds an M.S. in biology from East Stroudsburg University and a D.V.M. from the North Carolina State University's College of Veterinary Medicine, and has earned the R.A.C. (U.S.) certification.

# More About Selected Authors

**Meredith L. Huml** is a journalism student at Wake Technical Community College located in Wake County, North Carolina. Meredith previously served as a photographer and author during her tenure at Immaculata Catholic School (for *The Eagle Express*, her middle school's newspaper and yearbooks) and her high school, Cardinal Gibbons College Preparatory High School (for *The Crusader*, her school's newspaper).

Meredith currently works in graphic design, charcoal artwork, and writes poetry. She was diagnosed with FSHD in 2003 at Duke University's MDA Center.

**Jean K. Mah** is a pediatric neurologist and director of the Pediatric Neuromuscular Clinic at the Alberta Children's Hospital in Calgary, Alberta, Canada. She is an Associate Professor in the Department of Pediatrics and Clinical Neurosciences at the University of Calgary. She completed her Pediatrics training at the University of Alberta, her Neurology training at the University of North Carolina, her Neuromuscular fellowship at the Medical College of Virginia, and her Master of Science degree in Health Research from the University of Calgary. She has been a member of the Cooperative International Neuromuscular Research Group since 2005. Dr. Mah is currently involved in a number of collaborative research studies related to pediatric neuromuscular and demyelinating diseases.

**Kathryn R. Wagner, M.D., Ph.D.** is the Director of the Center for Genetic Muscle Disorders at the Kennedy Krieger Institute and Associate Professor of Neurology and Neuroscience at the Johns Hopkins School of Medicine. She treats patients with muscular dystrophies in an interdisciplinary clinic, addressing the multiple medical and social issues affecting these individuals and families. Dr. Wagner conducts clinical trials in muscular dystrophy including the first clinical trial of nonsense suppression in Duchenne and the first clinical trial of myostatin inhibition in adult muscular dystrophy. Dr. Wagner's laboratory focuses on developing methods to promote muscle regeneration. A major emphasis of her laboratory has been on modulating myostatin, an endogenous regulator of muscle. Dr. Wagner's laboratory has shown that inhibition of myostatin stimulates muscle stem cells, improving muscle regeneration while reducing fibrosis in animal models of muscular dystrophy. Current efforts include collaborations with industry to combine stem cell and pharmacological therapies for enhanced regeneration. She is an advisor for the FSH Society, Parent Project Muscular Dystrophy, and the TREAT-NMD Advisory Committee for Therapeutics.

# Abbreviations

| | |
|---|---|
| ACA | (Patient Protection and) Affordable Care Act of 2010 |
| AE | Adverse event |
| AFO | Ankle–foot–orthotic |
| BiPAP | Bilevel positive airway pressure |
| BMD | Becker's muscular dystrophy |
| CFR | Code of Federal Regulations |
| CHMP | (European Union) Committee for Medicinal Products for Human Use |
| CNM | Centronuclear myopathy |
| DM | Myotonic dystrophy |
| DMD | Duchenne muscular dystrophy |
| DNA | Deoxyribonucleic acid |
| DUX4 | Double homeobox protein 4 gene |
| EMA | European Medicines Agency |
| EMG | Electromyogram |
| ER | Emergency room |
| EU | European Union |
| FSH | Facioscapulohumeral MD |
| FSHD | Facioscapulohumeral MD |
| ICH | International Conference on Harmonization |
| ICU | Intensive care unit |
| IFSHD | Infantile FSHD |
| IND | Investigational New Drug (Application) |
| IRB | Institutional Review Board |
| KAFO | Knee–ankle–foot–orthotic |
| LCSW | Licensed Clinical Social Worker |
| LGMD | Limb girdle muscular dystrophy |
| LSCSW | Licensed Specialist Clinical Social Worker |
| MD | Muscular dystrophy |
| MDA | (U.S.) Muscular Dystrophy Association |

| | |
|---|---|
| MD CARE Act | Muscular Dystrophy Community Assistance, Research and Education (Act) |
| MTM | Myotubular myopathy |
| MRI | Magnetic resonance imaging |
| NINDS | National Institute of Neurological Disorders and Stroke |
| NMN | Neuromuscular network |
| OOPD | FDA's Office of Orphan Products Development |
| OPMD | Oculopharyngeal muscular dystrophy |
| PPMD | Parent Project Muscular Dystrophy |
| RNA | Ribonucleic acid |
| U.S. | United States of America |

# Chapter 1
# Introduction to Muscular Dystrophy

**Raymond A. Huml**

## Introduction

The proteins and structures of certain processes associated with muscular dystrophy (MD) are beginning to be elucidated by scientists based on recent advances in our understanding of genetics. MD is a group of diseases that are clinically manifested in patients as progressive muscle weakness with associated loss of mobility, agility, and body movements as a result of defects in genes for the production of muscle proteins that result in the death of muscle cells and tissue.

With these scientific advances, the number of potential pharmaceutical targets has increased, resulting in heightened interest in investment, partnership, and collaboration. For example, GlaxoSmithKline (GSK) recently announced its first discovery partnership with academia, with the Fred Hutchinson Cancer Center for the treatment of FSHD [1].

In addition, many companies pursing potential treatments for MD have advanced to the Phase II and Phase III stage of clinical drug development, and one product from PCT Therapeutics may be fully approved in 2015.

This advancement from PCT Therapeutics would be the first drug approved for the treatment of the Duchenne and Becker forms of muscular dystrophy (DMD and BMD), which are genetic disorders that develop primarily in boys. They are caused by different mutations in the gene for dystrophin, a protein that is important for maintaining normal muscle structure and function. Loss of dystrophin causes muscle fragility that leads to weakness and loss of walking ability during the childhood and teen years. Ataluren (to be marketed as Translarna™) is an orally delivered drug intended to overcome the effects of a specific type of mutation, called a nonsense mutation,

R.A. Huml, M.S., D.V.M., R.A.C. (✉)
Biosimilars Center of Excellence, Quintiles Inc., 4820 Emperor Boulevard, Durham, NC 27703, USA
e-mail: raymond.huml@quintiles.com

© Springer International Publishing Switzerland 2015
R.A. Huml (ed.), *Muscular Dystrophy*, DOI 10.1007/978-3-319-17362-7_1

which is the cause of DMD and BMD in approximately 10–15% of individuals with the disease [2]. A nonsense mutation is an abnormality in a sequence of DNA that results in a truncated, incomplete, and usually nonfunctional protein product.

To address the best way to study these potential treatments, the International Conference on Harmonization (ICH) communities responded by issuing limited draft guidance in Europe. The situation has similarities to that for biosimilars, where the European Union is ahead of the U.S. with regard to specific regulatory guidance. The European Medicines Agency (EMA) issued a concept paper in 2011 and, in early 2013, draft guidance for treatments related to DMD (and BMD). The U.S., on the other hand, appears to be relying on programs already in place to address the issues related to the potential treatment of MD. In 2013, when the U.S. Food and Drug Administration (FDA) addressed concerns from patient advocacy groups such as the Muscular Dystrophy Association (MDA), it cited existing programs to address the lack of specific MD regulatory guidance in the U.S. Programs specifically discussed included Fast Track Designation, Breakthrough Therapy Designation, Accelerated Approval and Priority Review [3].

This book provides an overview of MD with a focus on facioscapulohumeral MD (FSHD) in Chapter 3 and DMD and BMD in Chapter 4. Other forms of MD are presented and discussed, but not in as much detail, in Chapter 5. Later chapters, such as Chapter 11, examine some of the complex features that have made treatments for this group of diseases elusive. Chapter 10 provides an overview of the budding regulatory landscape for the treatment of MD in the EU and, finally, argues for more-detailed FDA guidance for each type of MD.

Lilleen Walters, who recently testified at a Congressional Briefing to reauthorize the Muscular Dystrophy CARE Act, said, "We must continue. If not us, then who? And if not now, then when? I believe that together, it's time to do something. With reauthorization and modest investments, we can restore a lot of smiles to a lot of people." It is important to note that Lilleen and her son, Collin, both have FSHD [4].

## Additional Support for Patients and Families with MD

Advocacy groups are discussed in greater detail in Chapter 13, titled, "U.S. Patient Advocacy Groups"; however, it is important to recognize that, as my father, Raymond G. Huml, Jr., used to say, that "each person is comprised of body, mind and *spirit*."

Indeed, in the June 25, 2014 letter from Pat Furlong to the FDA from the Parent Project Muscular Dystrophy, it is mentioned that each family, each parent of a child with DMD, has a different story to tell about their child's lifetime progressive loss of function, loss of independence, and dependence on family and the extraordinary burden—physically, financially, emotionally, and *spiritually*—that DMD places upon the caregiver and family [5].

When I led a group discussion of parents of children with FSHD at FSH Society's 2014 Biennial International Network Meeting in Boston, MA, several participants, including myself, cited their spiritual beliefs as providing comfort and a more hopeful perspective related to a diagnosis of FSHD.

Based on my opinion, all resources should be employed to support and encourage the MD patient and their family, including communities found within churches, synagogues, and other places of worship. It can be comforting to know that a group is praying for an afflicted family member and help/assistance can be as practical as obtaining a meal at a difficult time or assistance related to the healthcare needs of a family with a member afflicted with MD.

# References

1. Press release: Fred Hutchinson Cancer Research Center partners with GlaxoSmithKline to develop muscular dystrophy therapeutics. http://www.fredhutch.org/en/news/releases/2012/12/fred-hutch-gsk-partnership.html (2012). Accessed 7 Dec 2014.
2. Phase 2b Study of PTC124 in Duchenne/Becker Muscular Dystrophy (DMD/BMD). Clinical trials .gov website (2013). http://clinicaltrials.gov/ct2/show/NCT00592553?term=muscular+dystrophy&rank=5. Accessed 7 Dec 2014.
3. Temple RJ. Accelerated approval, Duchenne muscular dystrophy webinar. http://support.cure-duchenne.org/site/PageNavigator/FDAWebinar.html (2014). Accessed 7 Dec 2014.
4. Walters L. A lifetime of FSHD. A patient and mother speaks at congressional hearing, FSH Watch, Spring 2014. http://www.fshsociety.org/assets/pdf/FSHSociety_FSHWatch_Spring2014.pdf (2014). Accessed 30 May 2014
5. Duchenne Community Imperatives and Cover Letter—Draft Guidance on Duchenne. https://docs.google.com/file/d/0BznHl9zgmlY3WkhGY3VZaGZ3blk/edit?pli=1 (2014). Accessed 29 Aug 2014.

# Chapter 2
# Muscular Dystrophy: Historical Background and Types

Raymond A. Huml

## Historical Background

Reports vary, so there is no consensus as to who should be recognized as the first person to describe muscular dystrophy (MD). As Dr. Corrado Angelini rightly points out, "There is still controversy as to who should be given priority for the first description of MD." Further, he states that "The problem is confounded by the fact that it is now recognized that MD is not a single disease, but rather a heterogeneous set of diseases with different clinical phenotypes, pathological substrates, and both molecular and genetic determinants" [1].

According to the National Institute of Neurological Disorders and Stroke (NINDS) [2], the first historical accounts of MD appeared in 1830, when Sir Charles Bell (1774–1842) wrote an essay about an illness that caused progressive weakness in boys. Other sources point to Giovanni Semmola's publication in 1834 and later, a Semmola publication in conjunction with Gaetano Conte in 1836 [3].

The 1834 Semmola reference was his description of two boys affected by a previously undescribed disorder (in 1829), which he referred to as having the most noticeable sign of "muscular hypertrophy" [4].

According to Medscape [5], the first historical account of MD was given by Conte and Gioja in 1836 [6]. They described two brothers with progressive muscle weakness starting at age 10 and later developing generalized weakness and hypertrophy of multiple muscle groups, which are now known to be characteristic of the milder, Becker MD. At the time, however, many thought that Conte and Gioja were describing tuberculosis; thus, they did not achieve recognition for their discovery.

R.A. Huml, M.S., D.V.M., R.A.C. (✉)
Biosimilars Center of Excellence, Quintiles Inc., 4820 Emperor Boulevard,
Durham, NC 27703, USA
e-mail: raymond.huml@quintiles.com

© Springer International Publishing Switzerland 2015
R.A. Huml (ed.), *Muscular Dystrophy*, DOI 10.1007/978-3-319-17362-7_2

In 1852, Dr. Edward Meryon (1809–1880) reported a family with four boys, all of whom were affected by significant muscle changes, but no central nervous system abnormalities [7]. Meryon wrote a monograph on MD, suggesting a sarcolemmal defect as the cause of the disorder and suggesting that the disorder was genetically transmitted through females and affected only males.

The French neurologist, Guillaume Benjamin Amand Duchenne, MD (1806–1875), already famous for his use of electric currents to stimulate muscles and nerves, wrote about his first case of MD. In 1861, Duchenne described and detailed the case of boy who had DMD in his book titled, "Paraplegie hypertrophique de l'enfance de cause cerebrale" [8]. A year later, Duchenne presented photos of his patient in his "Album de photographes pathologiques." In 1868, he gave a comprehensive account of 13 patients with MD, which he called, "paralysie musculaire pseudo-hypertrophique ou paralysie myo-sclerosique." His descriptions of boys who grew progressively weaker, lost the ability to walk, and died at an early age became prominent in medical journals. Because Duchenne was already famous for his work with electrical stimulation, and later, for his contributions to the understanding of muscle disease, one of the most severe and well-known forms of MD, Duchenne MD, now bears his name.

Soon after DMD was identified, it became evident that more than one form of MD existed and that these diseases affected people of either gender and of all ages.

All of the MDs are inherited and involve a mutation in one of the thousands of genes that program proteins critical to muscle integrity and function. The muscle cells do not work properly when a protein is altered, produced in insufficient quantity, or missing. Many cases of MD occur from spontaneous mutations that are not found in the genes of either parent, and this defect can be passed on to the next generation.

MDs can be inherited in three ways: (1) autosomal inheritance (from a normal gene from one parent and an abnormal gene from another parent), (2) autosomal recessive inheritance (both parents carry and pass on the faulty gene), and (3) X-linked recessive inheritance (when a mother carries the affected gene and passes it on to her child).

Although MD can affect other body tissues and organs, it mostly affects the integrity of muscle fibers. The disease causes muscle degeneration, progressive weakness, fiber death, fiber branching and splitting, phagocytosis (in which muscle fiber is broken down and destroyed by scavenger cells) and, in some cases, chronic or permanent shortening of tendons and muscles. Overall muscle strength and tendon reflexes are usually lessened or lost due to replacement of muscle by connective tissue and fat.

## Other Types of MD

According to NIH's NINDS, there are nine major groups of MDs:

1. Duchenne MD
2. Becker MD
3. Congenital MD

4. Distal MD
5. Emery–Dreifuss MD
6. Facioscapulohumeral MD (FSHD)
7. Limb-girdle MD
8. Myotonic dystrophy (DM)
9. Oculopharyngeal MD (OPMD)

These disorders are characterized by the extent and distribution of muscle weakness, age of onset, rate of progression, severity of symptoms, and family history. Although some forms of MD appear in infancy or childhood, others may not appear until middle age or later. Overall, incidence rates vary, but each of the dystrophies causes progressive skeletal muscle deterioration.

Although it has been widely reported to be the third most common genetic disease of skeletal muscle, a 2008 analysis of rare diseases listed FSHD as the most prevalent form of MD at 7/100,000. This is discussed in greater detail in Chapter 3. DMD and BMD are discussed in Chapter 4 and the other MDs are discussed in Chapter 5.

# References

1. Angelini C. Muscular dystrophy. In: Chapter 31 in Handbook of clinical neurology, vol. 95. History of neurology. Amsterdam: Elsevier; 2009, p. 477–88.
2. Muscular dystrophy: hope through research, NIH's National Institute of Neurological Disorders and Stroke web site (2014). http://www.ninds.nih.gov/disorders/md/md.htm. Accessed 29 Aug 2014.
3. Nigro G. One-hundred-seventy-five years of Neapolitan contributions to the fight against the muscular diseases. Acta Myol. 2010;29(3):369–91. PMC 3146338 .
4. Semmola G. Sopra due malattie. Notizie dell'atra infermita. Acad Pontaniana. 1834; 164–5.
5. Do TT, chief editor. Medscape reference: drugs, diseases and procedures. muscular dystrophy; 2014. http://emedicine.medscape.com/article/1259041-overview. Accessed 29 Aug 2014.
6. Conte G, Gioja L. Scrofola del sistema muscolare. Ann Clin dell'Ospedale degli Incurabili Napoli. 1836;2:66–79.
7. Meryon E. On granular and fatty degeneration of the voluntary muscles. Med Chir Trans. 1852;35:73–4.
8. Duchenne GBA. Recherches sur la paralysie musculaire pseudo-hypertrophique ou paralysie myo-sclerosique. Arch Gen Med. 1868;11:5–25.

# Chapter 3
# FSHD: The Most Common Type of Muscular Dystrophy?

**Raymond A. Huml and Daniel P. Perez**

## Introduction

Facioscapulohumeral muscular dystrophy, a complex, inheritable muscle disease, was historically known as Landouzy–Déjérine disease—named after the French neurologists Dr. Joseph Jules Déjérine (1849–1917) and Dr. Louis Théophile Joseph Landouzy (1845–1917). It is more commonly known today as FSHD or FSH. Landouzy and Déjérine first named the disease FSHD in 1885 in order to distinguish the disease from the only other form of muscular dystrophy (MD) known at the time, DMD [1, 2].

Although frequently reported as the third most common type of MD in older reports and articles, many newer sources [3–5], including a May 2014 report by Orphanet, ranks FSHD as the most prevalent type of MD [6]. According to Orphanet, FSHD is the most prevalent MD with 7 cases/1,000 persons reported as compared with DMD/BMD (5 cases/1,000 persons) and Steinert myotonic dystrophy (4.5 cases/1,000 persons). Other prominent Websites, such as FSH Canada, also list FSHD as "the most prevalent of the nine primary types of MD affecting adults and children" [7]. Informal discussions with those afflicted with FSHD, as well as researchers and proponents of FSHD treatments, indicate that the incidence of FSHD is probably underreported. This may reflect the fact that some patients with FSHD—such as those with mild symptoms, or those with an onset late in life—may not ever be formally diagnosed and thus may not be reported or included in patient registries.

R.A. Huml, M.S., D.V.M., R.A.C. (✉)
Biosimilars Center of Excellence, Quintiles Inc., 4820 Emperor Boulevard, Durham, NC 27703, USA
e-mail: raymond.huml@quintiles.com

D.P. Perez
FSH Society, Inc., 450 Bedford Street, Lexington, MA 02420, USA

© Springer International Publishing Switzerland 2015
R.A. Huml (ed.), *Muscular Dystrophy*, DOI 10.1007/978-3-319-17362-7_3

The identification of FSHD as the most common type of MD has important ramifications, for example, when allocating future Federal (U.S.) funding for research. Daniel P. Perez, CEO and Founder of the FSH Society, has testified nearly 50 times before Congress. Due to his leadership efforts and testimony, funding for FSHD has grown from $1.5m/year in 2003 (out of $39.1m for all types of MD) to $5–6m in 2009–2013, a significant increase, but not yet aligned, based on prevalence alone. According to the most recent testimony by Mr. Perez to the U.S. Senate Appropriations Committee on May 16, 2014, FSHD is one of the most common adult MDs with a prevalence of 1:15,000–1:20,000 [6, 7].

Another important factor related to prevalence of disease is the potential market size for future FSHD treatments. Quite simply, a larger prevalence means a larger potential market and this may have an influence on the interest levels of third party capital providers investing in FSHD clinical trials and treatments. This is a win–win situation for both those afflicted with MD and those wishing to invest in the healthcare marketplace.

Despite being the most common form of MD, FSHD has only recently attracted attention from big pharma (e.g., GSK), largely due to major advances in the understanding of the gene/mechanism of disease [8]. For example, recent advances in the understanding of the cause of FSHD point to over-expression of a protein called DUX4, which is normally suppressed in adult muscles, but is activated in FSHD. A more detailed explanation is provided below in the section titled, "The Proposed Cause of FSHD."

## Overview of Symptoms of FSHD

The major symptom of FSHD is progressive weakening and loss of skeletal muscles. The usual location of these weaknesses at onset is the origin of the name: face (facio), shoulder girdle (scapulo), and upper arms (humeral). Early weaknesses of the muscles of the eye (open and close) and mouth (smile, pucker, whistle) are distinctive. These symptoms, in combination with weaknesses in the muscles that stabilize the scapulae (shoulder blades), are often the basis of the physician's clinical diagnosis of FSHD.

The progression of FSHD is quite variable, even among afflicted siblings [9]. For most patients, the progression of the disease is usually relatively slow; however, it usually worsens during adolescent years as the muscular framework fails to keep pace with the expanding and lengthening skeletal structure.

Other skeletal muscles invariably weaken. Involvement of muscles of the foot, hip girdle, and abdomen is common. With FSHD, most affected people develop unbalanced (side-to-side) weaknesses. The reason for this asymmetry is unknown [10].

In most cases, FSHD muscle involvement starts in the face and slowly progresses to the shoulder and upper-arm muscles and then down to the abdominal and foot-extensor muscles. Foot drop and foot weakness can be early manifestations and are generally accepted as part of the natural course of the disease [11, 12].

Initial signs of FSHD also include difficulty reaching above the shoulder level, scapular winging, and facial weakness. Weakness in the abdominal muscles can cause a protuberant abdomen and lumbar lordosis and scoliosis (curvatures of the lower spine). The inability to run and balance and loss of power may manifest in patients with FSHD and may be more noticeable in FSHD patients who play sports, take dance classes, or even school gymnastics classes, as FSHD patients compete with peers.

The lower abdominal muscles are usually weaker than the upper abdominal muscles. This distribution of weakness causes a positive Beevor's sign—a characteristic weakness of the lower abdominal muscles, involving the movement of the navel towards the head on flexing the neck—and, according to the FSH Society's Website and other sources [13], prognostic for FSHD.

Other symptoms in FSHD patients include chronic pain in the majority of patients (50–80%) with severe pain in up to 23% [14–16], vision abnormalities (due to vascular abnormalities of blood vessels in the back of the eye, which cause visual problems in only about 1% of the cases) [13], progressive hearing loss (correlated with the severity of genetic abnormalities and especially in severe infantile cases), cardiac arrhythmias (generally asymptomatic), and cognitive impairment, sometimes with epilepsy. The latter conditions are rare, but may be seen in severe, early-onset cases.

## Autosomal Dominance

Most individuals with FSHD inherit the mutation from a parent with the disease. DNA is the means of transmission of inheritable traits from parent to child and occurs via chromosome transfer from one generation to the next. Each chromosome contains a strand of DNA. Human cells usually contain 46 chromosomes, 23 from each parent. Children inherit one member of each of the 23 pairs of chromosomes from each parent. Forty-four of the chromosomes, also called autosomes, are homologous pairs (numbered 1 through 22), with each strand of the pair having the same size, order, and arrangement with genes for the same traits in the same position on the chromosome. The remaining chromosome pair consists of the nonhomologous sex chromosomes X and Y. A mother donates an X chromosome, and a father donates either an X or Y chromosome. Therefore, males have one X chromosome and one Y chromosome, while females have two X chromosomes [17].

FSHD is the result of a DNA mutation on one member of the chromosome 4 pair. FSHD is highly penetrant. This means that when a person inherits a chromosome 4 with the FSHD mutation, there is a high probability that discernible muscle weaknesses will develop. Since weakness still occurs in the presence of the normal member of the chromosome 4 pair, the disease is considered dominant. FSHD is, therefore, a dominant inherited disease, meaning only one parent has to have the disease gene or deletion for his or her child to inherit FSHD. Since each parent donates only one member of each chromosome pair to a child, the probability of passing the disease to an offspring is 50%.

If one has a blood parent, sibling, or other relative who has the FSHD mutation, there may be a risk of carrying that mutation. Often, when a person is diagnosed with FSHD, the disease is discovered to be throughout the extended family tree and over many generations. It is important to be aware that there may be other family members who are affected but unaware that they may have FSHD or may be at risk for FSHD. Professionals with knowledge of genetics and inheritance of FSHD can advise them regarding that risk.

## The Proposed Cause of FSHD

A DNA mutation causes FSHD. The gene that is linked to FSHD is unknown, but its approximate location is toward the end of the DNA of the long arm of chromosome 4. The specific genetic location of the FSHD deletion is 4q35 in the D4Z4 DNA region. Although the precise details are not yet known, the most probable cause of FSHD is inappropriate expression of protein called DUX4 by a "double homeobox protein 4 gene" [18, 19]. According to the FSH Society's Website, approximately 2% of FSHD cases are not linked to the 4q35 deletion on chromosome 4.

Researchers are investigating the molecular connection between deletion and FSHD. The size of the deletion has a relationship to the severity of the disease— patients with the fewest repeats (the largest deletion) typically have the most severe symptoms.

The DUX4 gene is normally expressed in germ line tissue (cells associated with reproduction, such as sperm and ovaries) and repressed in somatic cells (non-germ cells associated with forming other parts of the human body), but becomes over-expressed in FSHD patients and is toxic to muscle cells.

Two forms of the disease are recognized and reported in the literature: FSHD1 and FSHD2. About 95% of patients with FSHD have the FSHD1 form, where one allele (called D4Z4) is contracted and the other D4Z4 allele is normal [20, 21]. De novo, or sporadic contraction of D4Z4, account for 10–30% of FSHD1 cases [22, 23].

Less than 5% of FSHD patients have no contracted D4Z4 repeat arrays, but may still have abnormal DNA and are termed FSHD2 cases [24]. Patients with FSHD2 sometimes have another mutated gene, called SMCHD1, which appears to upregulate D4Z4 and be the cause of some, if not most, cases of FSHD2 [25]. There is no generally accepted estimate of its incidence, but this is unlikely to exceed 2% of all cases of FSHD.

Infantile FSHD (IFSHD) is characterized by onset in early childhood. There is no generally accepted estimate of its incidence, but it is rare. FSHD occurs in all racial groups and with equal frequency in both sexes.

One cannot clinically distinguish one type of FSHD from the other.

# De Novo Cases of FSHD [19]

Studies report from 10% to as high as 33% of all FSHD cases result from a de novo (or sporadic) mutation. Approximately 20% of reported de novo cases are those inherited from a seemingly unaffected parent who is a "germline mosaic," meaning that only the mother's or father's germ cells (the egg or sperm) are affected. When a germline mosaic is involved, the parent appears unaffected but the children are at risk.

In the remaining 80% of de novo cases, neither parent's genes are affected; a new spontaneous mutation results in a chromosome 4 deletion that causes FSHD. When the 4q35 deletion fragment appears in a sporadic FSHD case, it is transmitted in an autosomal dominant (only one parent needs to be affected) manner to succeeding generations. The probability, then, of passing the disease to an offspring is 50%.

# Onset of Symptoms

Although the FSHD gene is present at birth, weaknesses are generally not noticeable until the second decade. Sometimes, muscle weaknesses are slight throughout adulthood. A physician can usually clinically recognize and diagnose FSHD beyond the age of 20. However, it is important to realize that the onset of FSHD is highly variable and may require several physicians, with differing specialties, to diagnose younger patients or patients with milder symptoms.

In IFSHD, a young child or an infant develops symptoms. In IFSHD, there are facial weaknesses during the first two years of life in addition to other typical muscle weaknesses of FSHD. Some of these children also experience early hearing losses and retinal abnormalities.

# Prognosis of FSHD

Predicting the exact course and outcome of FSHD is impossible because the rapidity and extent of muscle loss differs considerably among FSHD patients—even among siblings. Some report few difficulties throughout life, while others need orthotic devices (e.g., abdominal brace, leg or foot braces) or a wheelchair as walking becomes difficult or impossible. The degree of severity in an FSHD parent cannot accurately predict the extent of disability that may develop in that parent's child.

Some reports suggest than men with FSHD are more severely affected than women [26, 27].

There is certainty that some skeletal muscles will weaken and waste throughout life and that this can, and often does, cause limitations on personal and occupational activities. The heart and internal (smooth) muscles seem spared and, with rare exceptions, those with FSHD have a normal life span.

## Diagnosing FSHD

Physical examinations by clinicians familiar with the disease, such as neurologists associated with an Muscular Dystrophy Association (MDA) Center, are dependable when there are clinical symptoms that follow an expected location and pattern of weakening muscles.

Often the physician will supplement a physical examination with inquiries about a possible family history of FSHD and may wish to take blood samples to help make the diagnosis. Other diagnostic tools that a physician may employ to confirm a diagnosis of FSHD include:

- Measurement of specific enzyme levels in the blood (e.g., creatine kinase or CK).
- An electromyograph or EMG, which records abnormal electrical activity of a functioning skeletal muscle.
- A muscle biopsy, where a small piece of muscle tissue is analyzed for visible abnormalities by a histopathologist.
- A DNA test, especially for equivocal cases for patients at younger ages and some at-risk adults with mild or asymptomatic cases. This test is highly reliable for most cases.
  - The test detects the 4q35 DNA deletion described earlier. Although several factors may occasionally complicate the test, the FSH Society states that confirmation of the 4q35 deletion is 98% reliable as a presumptive diagnosis of FSHD. The test requires no more than a small amount of blood that one's physician sends to a testing laboratory. The laboratory extracts sufficient DNA for the test from the cells present in the blood.
  - Currently, there is no DNA test available for those cases where there is no linkage between FSHD and chromosome 4.
- Prenatal testing, which is available for those persons interested.

Many physicians will also refer a patient diagnosed with FSHD to undergo further testing that may include:

- A visual exam, including a retinal examination
- Pulmonary function tests
- Cardiac tests
- Orthopedic examination
- Radiographic examination (especially for scoliosis and lordosis to determine a baseline and to monitor progression)
- Referral for physical therapy
- Orthotic (man-made support devices, usually made of cloth, plastic, or rubber) to support the abdomen (e.g., with lordosis) or extremities (e.g., foot drop)
- Measurements for assisted mobility devices, such as a scooter, Segway-type of device, or electronic wheelchair

Neurologists are often the primary physicians in muscle disease clinics since muscles do their work through stimulation by nerves. Physiatrists are physicians who work with chronic neuromuscular conditions. Periodic visits with a neurologist or physiatrist are useful to monitor the progress of FSHD and to obtain referrals to other professionals and services. An orthopedist (a physician concerned with the skeletal system and associated muscles, joints, and ligaments) can offer advice about mobility issues and other functional problems of the muscular/skeletal system. Those with experience in MD/FSHD are generally the most helpful.

Physical therapy, including light exercise, helps preserve flexibility. Swimming is especially helpful in this regard because of buoyancy and may make movements easier. According to the FSH Society's website, a patient with FSHD should stay as active as possible, with rest breaks as needed during exercise and activities.

Occupational therapists can help with suggestions for adaptations and physical aids that can often partially free an FSHD patient from some constrictions of the disease. Foot drop can sometimes be managed with ankle-foot orthotics (AFOs) and knee-ankle-foot orthotics (KAFOs). Occupational and ergonomic therapists may even visit a FSHD patient's home and make recommendations to improve the way a patient with FSHD can navigate their house or room.

Speech and hearing therapists can help with limitations imposed by hearing loss and weakened facial musculature to improve speech and communication.

## Psychiatry and Psychological Counseling

While it is beyond the scope of this chapter to delve into all of the facets of psychiatric and psychological counseling for patients afflicted with FSHD, suffice it to say that a diagnosis of FSHD can be devastating to the patient, the patient's family, and the patient's caregivers. A patient, if diagnosed with clinical depression by a physician, may benefit from medication (e.g., antidepressants) and regular counseling sessions. This is not inexpensive, but may be covered, at least in part, by insurance carriers, though there is usually a cost difference between in-network (physicians who may or may not be familiar with MD) and out-of-network physicians (who could be those who are most familiar with MD or those most sought after, but may or may not be in the insurance carrier's plan).

There are many different types of experts who can provide counseling services for patients with FSHD; however, for simplicity, three are described below:

- A psychiatrist, a medically trained physician trained to treat mental disorders, can prescribe medication, if needed, to a patient with FSHD.
- A psychologist (e.g., Ph.D.), trained to understand mental disorders, can help a patient learn new skills required to cope with complex, life-altering diseases such as FSHD. These experts cannot prescribe medication, but typically cost less per hour than psychiatrists.
- A Licensed Specialist Clinical Social Worker (LSCSW) or Licensed Clinical Social Worker (LCSW), with a Master's degree in Social Work plus supervised experience and the required amount of continuing education, can counsel patients and families with FSHD and typically cost less than psychologists and psychiatrists.

## Treatments for FSHD

There is currently no disease modifying treatment or cure for FSHD. Most treatments currently considered or proposed to "treat" FSHD have not yet been tested in randomized clinical trials. These may include: hormone supplementation (e.g., testosterone), protein supplements (creatinine monohydrate), or drugs used to decrease inflammation (e.g., prednisone). To better understand and validate their use, many are now being properly investigated in clinical trials. See paragraph below titled, "Clinical Trials for Patients with FSHD" for additional details.

Pain is part of FSHD in many patients. No specific treatments are available. Pain medication and mild physiotherapy are often prescribed with moderate results.

Sometimes an orthopedic surgeon may recommend attaching the scapulae (shoulder blades) to the back to improve motion of the arms. An individual who is considering such surgery should consult with their neurologist or physiatrist and an orthopedic surgeon. Discussion of this procedure with individuals who have undergone the surgery is highly recommended.

Sometimes an orthopedic surgeon may wish to fuse the spinal column of a FSHD patient in order to correct lordosis/scoliosis. As this surgery is rarely performed, an individual may wish to consult with their neurologist, physiatrist, or other orthopedic/pediatric surgeons to determine possible negative or untoward consequences. Because this surgery may decrease or eliminate compensatory mechanisms and decrease remaining ambulatory time for a patient with FSHD, it is advisable to obtain several professional opinions to understand the risks and benefits of such a surgery before deciding upon this type of surgery for an ambulatory patient with FSHD.

Further discussion of treatment for patients with MD, not exclusively for FSHD, is provided in Chapter 7.

## Mobility Devices for Patients with FSHD

If a FSHD patient requires a mobility device, such as an electronic wheelchair (usually due to fatigue associated with walking or the inability to walk) or scooter, there is an extensive and sometimes protracted process that a patient must undergo to satisfy insurance requirements justifying their use and procurement. Based on the author's experience, time limitations exist for physicians seeking to obtain a wheelchair for their FSHD patient (e.g., the physician recommending the procurement of a wheelchair must have seen the FSHD patient within the last six months) and may be limited to physicians practicing in the patient's state of residence. This can be difficult for patients with FSHD who seek optimum treatment and may need to travel out of state to visit a physician or may have visited a physician within their state, but not within the six month "statute of limitations." Therefore, the patient with FSHD and his/her caregiver should seek the advice of mobility provider to make sure that the initial application has the highest probability of success upon initial submission/request. NuMotion, a provider of wheelchairs in North Carolina (and a hub for the MDA "closet" where devices for persons afflicted with MD are offered for free), is one example of a mobility provider that not only understands the situation for families dealing with MD, but can act as an advocate for the entire family.

The MDA can be helpful in assisting patients with FSHD or even provide loaner wheelchairs—called "closet wheelchairs"—free of charge for those that qualify or for patients waiting for a customized wheelchair. There may be assistance regarding their upkeep and repair, and patients and caregivers should inquire about such services when procuring a wheelchair. It is beyond the scope of this chapter to discuss mobility transport, but it may include: wheelchair with ramps to place the wheelchair in a van/truck; exterior carriers that mount to a hitch on the back of a vehicle; and collapsible scooters that can be taken apart to carry in the trunk of a car.

## Clinical Trials for Patients with FSHD

*Clinicaltrials.gov* lists 17 trials using the search term "FSHD", but this may be a little misleading as the 17th trial (as accessed on June 2, 2014) actually lists the title of the trial as for DMD and not FSHD. Most of the trials posted are related to the study of antioxidants, protein supplementation, and physical therapy and may be out of date or abandoned for lack of efficacy or the inability to obtain additional funding. Some of the compounds under investigation, such as albuterol and prednisone, have been marketed for many years, but are not approved for FSHD, and therefore, have not been formally studied in the clinical trial setting for the treatment of FSHD. Some products, at first blush, appear to be unique, such as Wyeth's (now Pfizer's) MYO-029; however, the last update was in 2007 and the Website states that the trial is now closed. A review of ADIS reports (in June 2014) lists MYO-029 as "discontinued in Phase II."

Additional discussion of treatments, including a discussion of clinical trials, is provided in Chapter 12.

## FSHD Respiratory Insufficiency [10]

Respiratory involvement may be seen with FSHD. Evaluation of the symptoms and signs of respiratory insufficiency should be sought during routine clinic visits in patients with moderate to severe FSHD. Regular monitoring of respiratory function is suggested as individuals might experience insufficiency over a long period of time without presenting signs.

Symptomatic respiratory insufficiency can be initially managed with nighttime noninvasive pressure support, e.g., a BiPAP machine. In very severe cases, patients may require the use of a ventilator. For FSHD patients with respiratory insufficiency, in standard practice, trauma (ER, ICU), surgery, and anesthesiology settings, care should be taken not to suppress respiratory drive with narcotics unless it is a situation of palliative care. It is important to notify the doctors about FSHD and any respiratory problems the patient might have or be at risk for.

Oxygen supplementation can be detrimental to patients with hypercarbic (high $CO_2$) respiratory failure and lead to worsening $CO_2$ levels. Oxygen should generally not be administered unless BiPAP or similar ventilatory support is also being used. Consultation with the patient's primary physician and a pulmonologist can enable periodic monitoring of $CO_2$ levels in the office/school setting or pulmonary function lab in the hospital.

# References

1. Landouzy L, Déjérine J. De la myopathie atrophique progressive. Rev Med. 1885;5:81–117, 253–366.
2. Upadhyaya M, Cooper DN, editors. FSHD, facioscapulohumeral muscular dystrophy: clinical medicine and molecular cell biology. London: BIOS Scientific Publishers; 2004; ISBN: 18599 62440.
3. Facts and Statistics about FSHD. University of Massachusetts Medical School. http://www.umassmed.edu/wellstone/aboutfshd/FSHDfacts/. Accessed 11 Jun 2014.
4. Flanigan KM, et al. Genetic characterization of a large, historically significant Utah kindred with facioscapulohumeral muscular dystrophy. Neuromuscul Disord. 2001;11:525–9.
5. Mostacciuolo ML, et al. Facioscapulohumeral muscular dystrophy: epidemiological molecular study in a north-east Italian population sample. Clin Genet. 2009;75:550–5.
6. Prevalence of rare diseases: bibliographic data, www.orpha.net, May 2014 Number 1, Orphanet Report Series. http://www.orpha.net/orphacom/cahiers/docs/GB/Prevalence_of_rare_diseases_by_alphabetical_list.pdf. Accessed 30 May 2014.
7. FSHD Canada Foundation website. http://www.fshd.ca/what_overview.html. Accessed 9 June 2014.
8. Fred Hutchinson Cancer Research Center partners with GlaxoSmithKline to develop muscular dystrophy therapeutics. Newswise website. http://www.newswise.com/articles/fred-hutchinson-cancer-research-center-partners-with-glaxosmithkline-to-develop-muscular-dystrophy-therapeutics (2012). Accessed 25 Oct 2013.
9. Lunt PW, Harper PS. Genetic counseling in facioscapulohumeral muscular dystrophy. J Med Genet. 1991;28:655–64.
10. FSH Society website. http://www.fshsociety.org/pages/about.html. Accessed 23 May 2014.
11. Tyler FH, Stephens FE. Studies in disorders of muscle: II: clinical manifestations and inheritance of facioscapulohumeral muscular dystrophy in a large family. Ann Int Med. 1950;32:640–60.
12. Padberg GW. Facioscapulohumeral disease. Thesis, Leiden; 1982.
13. Darras BT. UptoDate: facioscapulohumeral muscular dystrophy. Wolters Kluwer Health; 2014, p. 16.
14. Van der Kooi EL, Kalkman JS, Linderman E, et al. Effects of training and albuterol on pain and fatigue in facioscapulohumeral muscular dystrophy. J Neurol. 2007;254:931.
15. Jensen MP, Hoffman AJ, Stoelb BL, et al. Chronic pain in persons with myotonic dystrophy and fasioscapulohumeral muscular dystrophy. Arch Phys Med Rehabil. 2008;89:320.
16. Padua L, Aprile I, Frusciante R, et al. Quality of life and pain in patients with facioscapulohumeral muscular dystrophy. Muscle Nerve. 2009;40:200.

17. Facts about genetics and neuromuscular diseases, copyrighted by the Muscular Dystrophy Association (MDA); 2011, p. 15.
18. Gabriels J, Beckers MC, Ding H, et al. Nucleotide sequence of the partially deleted D4Z4 locus in a patient with FSHD identifies a putative gene within each 3.3kb element. Gene. 1999;236:25.
19. Richards M, Coppee F, Thomas N, et al. Facioscalpulohumeral muscular dystrophy (FSHD): an enigma unraveled? Hum Genet. 2012;131:325.
20. Lemmers RJ, Miller DG, van der Maarel SM. Facioscapulohumeral muscular dystrophy. Gene Rev. http://www.ncbi.nlm.nih.gov/books/NBK1443/. Accessed 28 Jun 2014.
21. Stratland JM, Tawi R. Facioscapulohumeral muscular dystrophy: molecular pathological advances and future directions. Curr Opin Neurol. 2001;24:423.
22. Kohler J, Rupilius B, Otto M, et al. Germline mosaicism in 4q35 facioscapulohumeral muscular dystrophy (FSHD1A) occurring predominantely in oogenesis. Hum Genet. 1996;98:485.
23. Bakker E, Van der Wielen MJ, Voorhoeve E, et al. Diagnostic, predictive, and prenatal testing for facioscapulohumeral muscular dystrophy: diagnostic approach for sporadic and familial cases. J Med Genet. 1996;33:29.
24. van Overveld PG, Lemmers RJ, Sandkuijl LA, et al. Hypomethylation of D4Z4 in 4q-linked and non-4q-linked facioscapulohumeral muscular dystrophy. Nat Genet. 2003;35:315.
25. Lemmers RJ, Tawul R, Petek LM, et al. Digenic inheritance of an SMCHD1 mutation and an FSHD-permissive D4Z4 allele causes facioscapulohumeral muscular dystrophy type 2. Nat Genet. 2012;44:1370.
26. Zatz M, Marie SK, Cerqueira A, et al. The facioscapulohumeral muscular dystrophy (FSHD1) gene affects males more severely and more frequently than females. Am J Med Genet. 1998;77:155.
27. Tonini MM, Passos-Bueno MR, Cerqueira A, et al. Asymptomatic carriers and gender differences in facioscapulohumeral muscular dystrophy (FSHD). Neuromuscul Disord. 2004;14:33–8.

# Chapter 4
# Duchenne and Becker Muscular Dystrophies: Underlying Genetic and Molecular Mechanisms

Jean K. Mah

## Introduction

Duchenne and Becker muscular dystrophy are allelic disorders caused by mutations of the Duchenne muscular dystrophy (DMD) gene located on Xp21, which encodes for the dystrophin protein. DMD is the most common form of muscular dystrophy (MD) in childhood, with an estimated incidence of 1 per 3,500 live-born males [1] and a pooled prevalence of DMD of 4.78 (95% CI 1.94–11.81) per 100,000 males worldwide [2]. A brief review of the historical development serves to highlight the key clinical features associated with this disease. The condition was first described by Edward Meryon (1809–80), a British physician, in the 1850s [3]. His detailed clinical descriptions of eight affected boys including difficulty walking from an early age and later climbing stairs, with loss of ambulation and death occurring teenage years without any intervention are consistent with the progression and natural history of DMD. By microscopic exam, Meryon correctly surmised that the defect lies in the muscle cytoskeleton. A decade later, Duchenne described a young boy suffering from a progressive condition characterized by muscular weakness and calves hypertrophy; he was credited with the name for this disease [4]. In 1879, Gowers wrote a detailed review of the literature on DMD, including his own series of 20 cases. He provided clear illustrations of the method utilized by children with DMD to rise from the ground to a standing position; to this day, this phenomenon is still referred to as the Gowers' sign [5].

Becker muscular dystrophy (BMD) is a generally milder and more variable form of dystrophinopathy, with an incidence of 1 in 18,518 male births [1], and a pooled prevalence of 1.53 (95% CI 0.26–8.94) per 100,000 males worldwide [2].

J.K. Mah, M.D., M.Sc. (✉)
Department of Pediatrics and Clinical Neurosciences, University of Calgary,
Alberta Children's Hospital, 2888 Shaganappi Trail NW, Calgary, AB, Canada, T3B 6A8
e-mail: jean.mah@albertahealthservices.ca

© Springer International Publishing Switzerland 2015
R.A. Huml (ed.), *Muscular Dystrophy*, DOI 10.1007/978-3-319-17362-7_4

Similar to DMD, boys with BMD present with progressive muscle weakness and calf hypertrophy; however, the onset is often later and the progression is slower in BMD [6], with affected boys usually walking beyond the age of 16 years. Other presenting complaints of dystrophinopathies include myalgia and cramps [7], developmental delay, cognitive dysfunction [8], or dilated cardiomyopathy [9].

## Case Example

A two-year-old boy was referred for gross motor and speech delay. He was born at 36 weeks with a birth weight of 3.2 kg; there were no postnatal complications. He rolled at 6 months, sat at 12 months, and walked at 19 months of age. His speech was delayed, with only five words at two years. Family history was unremarkable. On examination his growth parameters were normal. Cranial nerves II to XII were intact. Motor exam revealed symmetrical bulk and tone, with prominent calf muscles. Spontaneous antigravity strength was present in all four limbs, but he needed help to get up from the floor. Deep tendon reflexes were 2+ throughout, with downgoing plantar responses. Sensation and gait were grossly intact. Investigations including brain MR imaging, TSH, hearing, and metabolic screen were normal. Serum creatine kinase (CK) levels were elevated, ranging from 7,975 to 17,988 U/L. Molecular genetic testing showed deletion of exons 46–53, an out-of-frame mutation in the dystrophin gene, consistent with a diagnosis of DMD.

In addition to motor developmental delay, proximal more than distal muscle weakness, and calf hypertrophy, this case illustrates that boys with DMD may have variable degrees of speech delay and/or cognitive impairment. Serum creatine kinase is usually markedly elevated, and muscle biopsy shows a dystrophic process with absent immunostaining for dystrophin. Progressive muscle degeneration is associated with scoliosis, cardiomyopathy, and respiratory insufficiency. With appropriate supportive strategies such as noninvasive positive pressure ventilation, survival beyond the third decade of life is now possible for many young adults with DMD [10, 11].

## Genetics

The DMD gene is one of the largest known human genes. It contains 79 exons, including an actin-binding domain at the N-terminus, 24 spectrin-like repeat units, a cysteine-rich dystroglycan binding site, and a C-terminal domain [12, 13]. The extremely large size of the gene contributes to a high spontaneous mutation rate [14]; approximately one-third of cases occur as a result of de novo mutations [15]. Two-thirds of DMD mutations are due to large deletions, while duplications occur in about 10% of cases; the remaining 25% include small deletions, insertions, point mutations, splicing mutations, as well as other complex mutational spectra [16, 17].

Details on dystrophin mutations are available from the Leiden muscular dystrophy database (www.dmd.nl). According to the reading frame hypothesis, the phenotype for the majority (90%) of dystrophinopathies can be predicted by whether the genetic alteration results in an in-frame or out-of-frame mutation [18]. In-frame mutations produce a semifunctional truncated dystrophin protein resulting in BMD, whereas DMD is the result of out-of-frame mutations leading to a severely truncated and non-functional protein [19]. Three full-length isoforms are derived from independent promotors in brain, retina, and Purkinje cerebellar neurons. These and other tissue-specific isoforms are responsible for the extramuscular manifestations, including cognitive and learning issues [20].

## Pathogenesis

Dystrophin is a 427 kDa cytoskeletal protein which is essential for muscle fiber stability. It binds to F-actin via its N-terminus and a cluster of basic repeats in its rod domain [20]. It also binds to dystroglycan via its cysteine-rich domain, and to dystrobrevin and syntrophin via its C-terminal domain; the latter is associated with nNOS, which is important in regulating the vasomotor response of the muscle, particularly during periods of exercise [21]. The dystrophin glycoprotein complex confers structural stability by forming a bridge across the sarcolemma and connecting the basal lamina of the extracellular matrix to the inner cytoskeleton; it is also essential for cell survival via its transmembrane signaling function [22]. Loss of dystrophin as a result of DMD gene mutations disrupts the dystrophin glycoprotein complex, leading to a cascade of events resulting in progressive muscle degeneration with diminished regenerative capacity, satellite cell depletion, and connective tissues replacement. In the absence of proper membrane-matrix attachment, mechanical stress from muscle contraction produces defects in the sarcolemma, with influx of calcium through the membranous lesions or through ion channels [21, 23]. Calcium dysregulation activates calcium-dependent proteases to further degrade muscle membrane proteins [24]. Furthermore, loss of nitric oxide results in increased oxidative stress, tissue ischemia, and reparative failure [25]. The progression is clearly visible with more severe fibrosis and fatty replacement, as well as more variation in fiber size in the later muscle biopsies [26].

## Diagnosis

The diagnosis of Duchenne and Becker muscular dystrophy is based on careful review of the clinical features and confirmed by additional investigations including muscle biopsy and/or genetic testing [27, 28]. Suspicion of the diagnosis of DMD is usually triggered in one of three ways, including (1) most commonly, the observation of abnormal muscle function with signs of proximal muscle weakness in a male child; (2) the detection of elevated serum creatine kinase as part of routine screening; or (3) the presence of elevated liver enzymes including aspartate aminotransferase and alanine aminotransferase, both of which are produced by muscle as well as liver cells. The presence of gross motor or speech delay in a male child should trigger the order of serum creatine kinase as initial diagnostic screening for DMD, especially if the child also has an abnormal gait [29]. A positive family history is not required as up to one-third of cases may occur as a result of spontaneous mutation.

Detection methods for DMD mutations include multiplex PCR that examines the most commonly deleted regions of the gene, and other assays that interrogate all 79 exons, such as the multiplex ligation-dependent probe amplification (MLPA) or comparative genomic hybridization (CGH) microarray [17, 30]. If the presence of a disease-causing deletion or duplication is not identified by a state-of-the-art DNA diagnostic technique, complete gene sequencing is helpful to define the precise mutational event. A muscle biopsy can also be obtained for dystrophin immunostaining plus extraction of cDNA and RNA. Using all available diagnostic methods, it is possible to identify the dystrophin mutations and confirm the clinical phenotypes in nearly all patients with dystrophinopathy [31]. Identification of a specific dystrophin mutation is important for accurate diagnosis, prognosis, and treatment for patients with DMD/BMD as well as genetic counseling for their families. Most heterozygous female carriers of DMD mutations are asymptomatic. Approximately 2–8% of these carriers are manifesting carriers (MCs) who develop mild to moderately severe progressive DMD-like muscular dystrophy [32–34]. Rarely, they can also present exclusively with cognitive and/or cardiac dysfunction [35].

## Treatment

There is presently no cure for DMD. Current strategies include promoting proper nutrition, delaying the onset of complications, and optimizing health outcomes through on-going support [27, 28]. Pharmaceutical interventions include the use of corticosteroids for skeletal muscle weakness and afterload reduction for cardiomyopathy. The introduction of noninvasive positive pressure ventilation has prolonged the survival of individuals with DMD. The mean age of death from DMD was 14.4 years in the 1960s, compared to 25.3 years since the advent of home ventilation in the 1990s, with improvement in patients' health-related quality of life [11, 36].

## *Therapeutic Strategies*

Recent scientific advances have led to potential disease modifying treatments for many neuromuscular diseases including DMD [37, 38]. Updated information about DMD clinical trials is available at http://www.clinicaltrials.gov. Treatments are also discussed in Chapters 7 and 12 of this book. Identification of coordination centers and patients eligible for specific DMD trials has been greatly facilitated by the establishment of TREAT-NMD and other international DMD disease registries [39]. The main therapeutic strategies include: (a) muscle membrane stabilization and upregulation of compensatory proteins [40, 41]; (b) enhancement of muscle regeneration and reduction of the inflammatory cascade [42, 43]; and (c) gene therapy to restore protein production [44, 45]. Examples of current therapeutic strategies are highlighted below.

## Gene Therapy

(a) Gene-replacement using virus vectors: Previous attempts to develop gene therapy for DMD have been complicated by the enormous size of the dystrophin gene. Subsequently, deletion of multiple regions of the dystrophin protein led to generation of highly functional mini- and micro-dystrophins; injection of adeno-associated viruses carrying micro-dystrophins into dystrophic muscles of canine model of DMD results in a striking improvement in the histopathological features of this disease [26, 46]. Clinical trials designed to replace defective genes in DMD are in progress [47].

(b) Exon-skipping: Exon-skipping uses synthetic antisense oligonucleotide sequences to correct the dystrophin gene deletion by causing the muscle cells to "skip over" the reading of specific exons, and then produce an internally truncated protein similar to the dystrophin protein expression seen in BMD. An earlier phase 1 clinical trial using PRO051, an antisense oligonucleotide, showed partial restoration of dystrophin after a single intramuscular injection into the tibialis anterior muscles of four boys with DMD [48]. This was followed by other phase 2 studies including repeated injections of drisapersen, a $2'$-$O$-methyl-phosphorothioate antisense oligonucleotide, into a larger number of DMD boys over a 48-week study period, with similar promising results [49]. Antisense therapies that induce single or multiple exon-skipping could potentially be helpful for other types of dystrophin mutations [50, 51].

(c) Nonsense suppression therapy: Approximately 10–15% of dystrophin mutation is due to point mutation leading to a premature stop codon [52]. Premature stop codons are nucleotide triplets within mRNA that signal the termination of translation by binding release factors which cause the ribosomal subunits to disassociate, releasing the amino acid chain, and causing any resulting protein to be abnormally shortened. This often results in a loss of function in the protein, as critical parts of the amino acid chain are no longer created. Ataluren, also known as PTC124, is an orally bio-available drug candidate designed to overcome premature nonsense mutations [53]. It binds to the large ribosomal subunit, where it causes a conformational change and thus allows ribosomes to read through the premature stop codon in mRNA to produce a modified dystrophin protein. Phase 2 and 3 studies of ataluren show promise for the treatment of boys with premature stop codon mutations [54, 55].

## Cellular Targets

(a) Cytoskeleton protein upregulation: The dystrophin glycoprotein complex forms a bridge across the sarcolemma and flexibly connects the basal lamina of the extracellular matrix to the inner cytoskeleton. It also acts as a transmembrane signaling complex which is essential for cell survival. Compensatory upregulation of cytoskeleton proteins including utrophin [56], alpha-7-beta-1 integrin [57], biglycan [58], and sarcospan [59] have been shown to stabilize the sarcolemma in the absence of dystrophin in mdx mice. Further clinical trials are pending.

(b) Nuclear factor-kappa B (NF-κB): In DMD mouse models and patients, the IκB kinase/NF-κB (IKK/NF-κB) signaling is persistently elevated in immune cells and regenerative muscle fibers [60]. As well, activators of NF-κB such as tumor necrosis factor-α (TNF-α) and interleukins (IL-1 and IL-6) are upregulated in DMD muscle. As pharmacological inhibition of NF-κB using the NEMO-binding domain (NBD) peptide resulted in improved pathology and muscle function in murine model of MD [61, 62], additional research is needed to identify the role of selective NF-κB modulators for use in DMD. Potential therapies include N-acetylcysteine [63], green tea extract [64], idebenone [65, 66], and melatonin [67, 68] for DMD.

## Muscle Regeneration

(a) Insulin-like growth factor (IGF-1): The therapeutic potential of upregulating a positive regulator of muscle development and regeneration using IGF-1 has been demonstrated in the dystrophic mouse models, especially when combined with mesenchymal stromal cells [69, 70]. Due to its regeneration-enhancing mechanism, this combinational approach may have general applicability for other MDs.

(b) Myostatin inhibition: Myostatin is a negative regulator of muscle mass. Inhibition or blockade of endogenous myostatin offers a potential means to compensate for the severe muscle wasting that is common in many types of MDs including DMD. A phase I/II multicenter clinical trial using a myostatin blocking antibody (MYO-029) for adult subjects with Becker muscular dystrophies and other dystrophies demonstrated safety, but was not sufficiently powered for efficacy [71]. Clinical trials using follistatin and other myostatin inhibitors are on-going [72, 73].

(c) Transforming growth factor-β (TGF-β): Elevated levels of TGF-β in MDs stimulate fibrosis and impair muscle regeneration by blocking the activation of satellite cells. A number of anti-fibrotic agents have been tested in murine models of MD, including losartan, an angiotensin II-type 1 receptor blocker that reduces the expression of TGF-β [74–76]. Other potential fibrosis inhibitors include halofuginone [77] and targeted microRNAs [78, 79]; further clinical trials are pending.

## *Standard of Care for DMD*

Until there is a cure, current treatment strategies for DMD focus on promoting well-balanced diet, participating in regular physical activity as tolerated, delaying the onset of complications via pharmaceutical treatments, and optimizing health outcomes through appropriate medical and psychosocial support. Recent publications have provided comprehensive reviews on the diagnosis and multidisciplinary management of DMD, including the use of prednisone or deflazacort (a corticosteroid anti-inflammatory product) to preserve muscle strength [80, 81], optimizing growth and development, surveillance for spinal deformities [82], managing respiratory complications [83, 84], and treating cardiomyopathy [85, 86]. As well, bone health, nutrition, learning disability, behavior problems, access to wheelchairs, and other adaptive technology should be included as part of the comprehensive treatment plan. The purpose of the DMD standard of care recommendations is to provide a framework for recognizing the primary manifestations and for planning optimum treatment across different specialties with a coordinated multidisciplinary team [27, 28]. Multidisciplinary coordination of care including respiratory, cardiac, orthopedic, and rehabilitative interventions has led to improvements in function, quality of life, health, and longevity.

Current pharmaceutical interventions include the use of corticosteroids for skeletal muscle weakness. Corticosteroids such as prednisone and deflazacort are the only medications currently available to fight against the rate of progression of muscle weakness and the development of secondary complications as part of the natural history of DMD. Deflazacort is an oxazoline derivative of prednisone, with similar side effects except for weight gain. Prednisone and deflazacort are being compared in a head-to-head fashion in the current FOR-DMD clinical trial. Historically, corticosteroids offer benefit to DMD boys by improving muscle strength and function [87, 88], prolonging independent ambulation [89, 90], plus slowing the progression of scoliosis [91] and cardiomyopathy [92]. On the basis of this literature and clinical experience, the current standard of care guideline strongly urge the consideration of corticosteroid therapy in all DMD patients [27, 28]. Continued treatment after the patient becomes non-ambulatory has also been shown to be beneficial [93].

A high index of suspicion for steroid-related side-effects needs to be maintained at all times, including the development of short stature, obesity, cataracts, and skeletal fractures [90, 94]. In particular, boys with DMD are at risk of developing multiple vertebral fractures due to combination of long-term corticosteroid use, muscular weakness, and immobility [95]. Given the impact of vertebral fractures on quality of life, cyclical intravenous pamidronate treatment should be considered to help minimize back pain and rebuild bone mass; however, long-term efficacy of bisphosphonate therapy for DMD remains limited [96, 97]. Current recommendation reserves the use of bisphosphonates to children with reduced bone mass plus symptomatic vertebral collapse and/or recurrent fragility fractures in the extremity, particularly in the context of persistent or multiple risk factors [27, 28].

Cardiac complication is common in DMD; most often it manifests as a cardiomyopathy and/or cardiac arrhythmia [98]. Cardiomyopathy is one of the leading causes of mortality in DMD [36, 99]. Despite the high prevalence of cardiac disease, most affected individuals are asymptomatic [100]; cardiac symptoms were reported in approximately 50% of DMD patients under 18 years of age, likely due to their low physical capability. Baseline assessment of cardiac function including electrocardiography (ECG) and echocardiogram should be done at diagnosis or by the age of six years, with reassessment at least once every two years until the age of ten years, and with annual complete cardiac assessments afterwards [27, 28]. Common ECG abnormalities include sinus tachycardia; as the posterior wall of the left ventricle is often most affected in DMD, abnormally tall R waves in V1 and deep Q waves in the inferolateral leads, ST depression, prolonged QT interval, and increased QT dispersion can also be found [101]. Echocardiographic evidence of structural heart disease in DMD patients includes LV hypertrophy, regional wall motion abnormalities, dilation of the cardiac chambers, valvular abnormalities, and LV systolic dysfunction [102]. Furthermore, LV wall motion abnormalities progress in a set sequence in DMD patients, initially involving the posterior wall and the apex, followed by the interventricular septum and finally the anterior wall [103]. Boys on corticosteroids will need additional monitoring for hypertension, especially when adjustment in the dose of corticosteroids is made periodically to compensate for growth. Afterload reduction therapy such as angiotensin-converting enzyme inhibitor or beta-blocker for cardiomyopathy may be indicated as early preventive treatment [27, 28, 101].

Patients with DMD are also at increasing risk of respiratory complications over time due to progressive loss of respiratory muscle strength. The earliest signs of respiratory insufficiency often manifest in sleep and include ineffective cough, nocturnal hypoventilation, sleep disordered breathing, and eventually daytime respiratory failure. Death is due to respiratory failure in the majority of individuals with DMD [36, 99]. The treatment of choice for sleep apnea and nocturnal hypoventilation in DMD patients is positive pressure ventilation, which can be delivered using nasal mask noninvasively. The use of noninvasive positive pressure ventilation has led to prolonged survival of individuals with DMD [104]. Benefits of noninvasive positive pressure ventilation include improved sleep quality, decreased daytime sleepiness, improved daytime gas exchange, and a slower decline in the pulmonary function, leading to reduced hospitalization and improved health-related quality of life. Additional supportive strategies may include mechanical insufflation–exsufflation and lung volume recruitment exercises [105, 106]. Treatment with oxygen alone should be avoided without ventilatory support as individuals with respiratory insufficiency secondary to DMD may develop worsening of their hypoventilation and hypercarbia [27, 28].

Individuals with DMD develop increasing joint contractures and loss of muscle extensibility as a result of progressive weakness, immobility, muscular imbalance about a joint, and fibrotic replacement in muscle tissue. Affected boys and their families should be taught how to do active, active-assisted, and/or passive stretching daily or at least of 4–6 days per week, initially focusing on the ankles and then to other joints or muscle groups as tolerated [27, 28]. Night splints can be worn to help minimize heel cord contractures, especially when present during the early ambulatory phase of DMD. Serial casting may also be tried for short periods of time as long as it does not significantly affect mobility [27, 28]. Ankle-foot-orthotics are generally not indicated for use during daytime ambulation as they may limit compensatory movements needed for efficient ambulation, add extra weight that can compromise ambulation, and make it difficult to rise from the floor [27, 28].

Routine health surveillance and meticulous growth record is important, especially for individuals with DMD in the pediatric age group. Anticipatory guidance including regular exercise, well-balanced diet, and avoidance of underweight/malnutrition or overweight/obese should be provided from diagnosis throughout life. The goal of optimal nutritional status, defined as weight for age or body-mass index for age from the 10th to 85th percentiles on national percentile charts, is encouraged [27, 28]. Referral to dietitian and more formal feeding or swallowing assessments may be indicated to help achieve these goals [107]. Other anticipatory guidance includes annual immunization with the trivalent inactivated influenza vaccine and periodic immunization with 23-valent pneumococcal polysaccharide vaccine is indicated, in addition to routine immunizations. Updates of recommendations are available through national organizations such as the American Academy of Pediatrics (www.aap.org) or the Centers for Disease Control and Prevention (www. cdc.gov/) in the U.S.

The medical care of individuals with DMD and their families requires multidisciplinary care and on-going psychosocial support. For many parents, the stress caused by the psychosocial problems of their child exceeds those associated with the physical aspects of the disease [108]. Increased burden of care and emotional distress are also common among caregivers of adults who have DMD [109]. These realities underscore the need for assessment and support of the entire family [27, 28]. Other parents learned to normalize their experience over time and experience similar levels of psychosocial stress to other families with healthy children [110, 111]. Indeed, there are both positive and negative experiences in living and caring for individuals with DMD [112]. One study provided parents of children with severe neuromuscular disease, such as DMD, the opportunity to speak of their daily lives and the challenges [110, 111]. The lived experience for the parents can be summed up by one keyword of being the "lifeline" for their child. However, this lifeline also embodies a reciprocal relationship with the child, as one parent explained: "I think it's more of a connection between the child and the parents are both lifelines for each other… you're receiving everything as much as you're giving." It challenges some of the assumptions about the disease, including the higher than expected quality of life and resilience shown by individuals with DMD and their families.

# Conclusion

The pathogenesis affecting DMD is complex; multiple interventions targeting different disease processes are needed. Early recognition and precise genetic diagnosis will allow for new emerging therapeutic options for DMD. Even though there is currently no cure, respiratory intervention and other supportive strategies as outlined in standard of care for DMD have led to improved survival and better health-related quality of life for many affected individuals. Those who are diagnosed today have the possibility of a life expectancy into their fourth decade. Collaboration remains the key strategy for optimizing neuromuscular care and advancing research for DMD globally.

# References

1. Emery AE. Population frequencies of inherited neuromuscular diseases—a world survey. Neuromuscul Disord. 1991;1(1):19–29.
2. Mah JK, Korngut L, Dykeman J, Day L, Pringsheim T, Jette N. A systematic review and meta-analysis on the epidemiology of Duchenne and Becker muscular dystrophy. Neuromuscul Disord. 2014;24(6):482–91.
3. Emery AE, Emery ML. Edward Meryon (1809–1880) and muscular dystrophy. J Med Genet. 1993;30(6):506–11.
4. Rondot PG. Duchenne de boulogne (1806–1875). J Neurol. 2005;252:866–7.
5. Kaya Y, Sarikcioglu L. Sir William Richard Gowers (1845–1915) and his eponym. Childs Nerv Syst. 2014.
6. Hoffman EP, Kunkel LM, Angelini C, Clarke A, Johnson M, Harris JB. Improved diagnosis of Becker muscular dystrophy by dystrophin testing. Neurology. 1989;39:1011–7.
7. Gospe Jr SM, Lazaro RP, Lava NS, Grootscholten PM, Scott MO, Fischbeck KH. Familial X-linked myalgia and cramps: a nonprogressive myopathy associated with a deletion in the dystrophin gene. Neurology. 1989;39:1277–80.
8. North KN, Miller G, Iannaccone ST, et al. Cognitive dysfunction as the major presenting feature of Becker's muscular dystrophy. Neurology. 1996;46:461–5.
9. Feng J, Yan J, Buzin CH, Towbin JA, Sommer SS. Mutations in the dystrophin gene are associated with sporadic dilated cardiomyopathy. Mol Genet Metab. 2002;77:119–26.
10. Center for Disease Control. Survival of males diagnosed with Duchenne/Becker muscular dystrophy (DBMD) by years of birth—Muscular Dystrophy Surveillance Tracking and Research Network. MMWR Morb Mortal Wkly Rep. 2009;58(40):1119–22.
11. Villanova M, Brancalion B, Mehta AD. Duchenne muscular dystrophy: life prolongation by noninvasive ventilatory support. Am J Phys Med Rehabil. 2014;93(7):595–9.
12. Hoffman EP, Brown RH, Kunkel LM. Dystrophin: the protein product of the Duchenne muscular dystrophy locus. Cell. 1987;51(6):919–28.
13. Koenig M, Monaco AP, Kunkel LM. The complete sequence of dystrophin predicts a rod-shaped cytoskeletal protein. Cell. 1988;53(2):219–28.
14. Aartsma-Rus A, Van Deutekom JC, Fokkema IF, Van Ommen GJ, Den Dunnen JT. Entries in the Leiden Duchenne muscular dystrophy mutation database: an overview of mutation types and paradoxical cases that confirm the reading-frame rule. Muscle Nerve. 2006;34(2):135–44.
15. Laing NG. Molecular genetics and genetic counselling for Duchenne/Becker muscular dystrophy. In: Partridge TA, editor. Molecular and cell biology of muscular dystrophy. London: Chapman & Hall; 1993. p. 37–84.

16. Mah JK, Selby K, Campbell C, Nadeau A, Tarnopolsky M, McCormick A, et al. A population-based study of dystrophin mutations in Canada. Can J Neurol Sci. 2011;38(3):465–74.

17. Nallamilli BR, Ankala A, Hegde M. Molecular diagnosis of Duchenne muscular dystrophy. Curr Protoc Hum Genet. 2014;83:9.25.1–29.

18. Monaco AP, Bertelson CJ, Colletti-Feener C, Kunkel LM. Localization and cloning of Xp21 deletion breakpoints involved in muscular dystrophy. Hum Genet. 1987;75(3):221–7.

19. Koenig M, Beggs AH, Moyer M, et al. The molecular basis for Duchenne versus Becker muscular dystrophy: correlation of severity with type of deletion. Am J Hum Genet. 1989;45(4):498–506.

20. Muntoni F, Torelli S, Ferlini A. Dystrophin and mutations: one gene, several proteins, multiple phenotypes. Lancet Neurol. 2003;2(12):731–40.

21. Wallace GQ, McNally EM. Mechanisms of muscle degeneration, regeneration, and repair in the muscular dystrophies. Annu Rev Physiol. 2009;71:37–57.

22. Amann KJ, Guo AW, Ervasti JM. Utrophin lacks the rod domain actin binding activity of dystrophin. J Biol Chem. 1999;274:35375–80.

23. Gumerson JD, Michele DE. The dystrophin-glycoprotein complex in the prevention of muscle damage. J Biomed Biotechnol. 2011;2011:210797.

24. Allen DG, Gervasio OL, Yeung EW, Whitehead NP. Calcium and the damage pathways in muscular dystrophy. Can J Physiol Pharmacol. 2010;88(2):83–91.

25. Thomas GD. Functional muscle ischemia in Duchenne and Becker muscular dystrophy. Front Physiol. 2013;4:381.

26. Shin J, Tajrishi MM, Ogura Y, Kumar A. Wasting mechanisms in muscular dystrophy. Int J Biochem Cell Biol. 2013;45(10):2266–79.

27. Bushby K, Finkel R, Birnkrant DJ, Case LE, Clemens PR, Cripe L, et al. Diagnosis and management of Duchenne muscular dystrophy, part 1: diagnosis, and pharmacological and psychosocial management. Lancet Neurol. 2010;9(1):77–93.

28. Bushby K, Finkel R, Birnkrant DJ, Case LE, Clemens PR, Cripe L, et al. Diagnosis and management of Duchenne muscular dystrophy, part 2: implementation of multidisciplinary care. Lancet Neurol. 2010;9(2):177–89.

29. van Ruiten HJ, Straub V, Bushby K, Guglieri M. Improving recognition of Duchenne muscular dystrophy: a retrospective case note review. Arch Dis Child. 2014;99(12):1074–7.

30. Hedge MR, Chin ELH, Mulle JG, Okou DT, Warren ST, Zwick ME. Microarray-based mutation detection in the dystrophin gene. Hum Mutat. 2008;29(9):1091–9.

31. Takeshima Y, Yagi M, Okizuka Y, Awano H, Zhang Z, Yamauchi Y, et al. Mutation spectrum of the dystrophin gene in 442 Duchenne/Becker muscular dystrophy cases from one Japanese referral center. J Hum Genet. 2010;55(6):379–88.

32. Moser H, Emery AE. The manifesting carrier in Duchenne muscular dystrophy. Clin Genet. 1974;5:271–84.

33. Norman A, Harper P. A survey of manifesting carriers of Duchenne and Becker muscular dystrophy in Wales. Clin Genet. 1989;36:31–7.

34. Taylor PJ, Maroulis S, Mullan GL, et al. Measurement of the clinical utility of a combined mutation detection protocol in carriers of Duchenne and Becker muscular dystrophy. J Med Genet. 2007;44:368–72.

35. Soltanzadeh P, Friez MJ, Dunn D, et al. Clinical and genetic characterization of manifesting carriers of DMD mutations. Neuromuscul Disord. 2010;20:499–504.

36. Eagle M, Baudouin SV, Chandler C, Giddings DR, Bullock R, Bushby K. Survival in Duchenne muscular dystrophy: improvements in life expectancy since 1967 and the impact of home nocturnal ventilation. Neuromuscul Disord. 2002;12(10):926–9.

37. Wagner KR. Approaching a new age in DMD treatment. Neurotherapeutics. 2008;5(4):583–91.

38. Mercuri E, Muntoni F. Muscular dystrophy: new challenges and review of the current clinical trials. Curr Opin Pediatr. 2013;25(6):701–7.

39. Bladen CL, Rafferty K, Straub V, Monges S, Moresco A, Dawkins H, et al. The TREAT-NMD Duchenne muscular dystrophy registries: conception, design, and utilization by industry and academia. Hum Mutat. 2013;34(11):1449–57.

40. Malik V, Rodino-Klapac LR, Mendell JR. Emerging drugs for Duchenne muscular dystrophy. Expert Opin Emerg Drugs. 2012;17(2):261–77.
41. Marshall JL, Crosbie-Watson RH. Sarcospan: a small protein with large potential for Duchenne muscular dystrophy. Skelet Muscle. 2013;3(1):1.
42. De Paepe B, De Bleecker JL. Cytokines and chemokines as regulators of skeletal muscle inflammation: presenting the case of Duchenne muscular dystrophy. Mediators Inflamm. 2013;2013:540370.
43. Motohashi N, Asakura A. Muscle satellite cell heterogeneity and self-renewal. Front Cell Dev Biol. 2014;2:1.
44. Konieczny P, Swiderski K, Chamberlain JS. Gene and cell-mediated therapies for muscular dystrophy. Muscle Nerve. 2013;47(5):649–63.
45. Bertoni C. Emerging gene editing strategies for Duchenne muscular dystrophy targeting stem cells. Front Physiol. 2014;5:148.
46. Shin JH, Pan X, Hakim CH, Yang HT, Yue Y, Zhang K, et al. Microdystrophin ameliorates muscular dystrophy in the canine model of Duchenne muscular dystrophy. Mol Ther. 2013;21(4):750–7.
47. Okada T, Takeda S. Current challenges and future directions in recombinant AAV-mediated gene therapy of Duchenne muscular dystrophy. Pharmaceuticals (Basel). 2013;6(7):813–36.
48. van Deutekom JC, Janson AA, Ginjaar IB, et al. Local dystrophin restoration with antisense oligonucleotide PRO051. N Engl J Med. 2007;357(26):2677–86.
49. Voit T, Topaloglu H, Straub V, Muntoni F, Deconinck N, Campion G, et al. Safety and efficacy of drisapersen for the treatment of Duchenne muscular dystrophy (DEMAND II): an exploratory, randomised, placebo-controlled phase 2 study. Lancet Neurol. 2014;13(10):987–96.
50. Aoki Y, Yokota T, Wood MJ. Development of multiexon skipping antisense oligonucleotide therapy for Duchenne muscular dystrophy. Biomed Res Int. 2013;2013:402369.
51. Al-Zaidy S, Rodino-Klapac L, Mendell JR. Gene therapy for muscular dystrophy: moving the field forward. Pediatr Neurol. 2014;51(5):607–18.
52. Finkel RS. Read-through strategies for suppression of nonsense mutations in Duchenne/Becker muscular dystrophy: aminoglycosides and ataluren (PTC124). J Child Neurol. 2010;25(9):1158–64.
53. Welch EM, Barton ER, Zhuo J, et al. PTC124 targets genetic disorders caused by nonsense mutations. Nature. 2007;447(7140):87–91.
54. Finkel RS, Flanigan KM, Wong B, Bönnemann C, Sampson J, Sweeney HL, et al. Phase 2a study of ataluren-mediated dystrophin production in patients with nonsense mutation Duchenne muscular dystrophy. PLoS One. 2013;8(12):e81302.
55. Bushby K, Finkel R, Wong B, Barohn R, Campbell C, Comi GP, et al. Ataluren treatment of patients with nonsense mutation dystrophinopathy. Muscle Nerve. 2014;50(4):477–87.
56. Tinsley JM, Fairclough RJ, Storer R, Wilkes FJ, Potter AC, Squire SE, et al. Daily treatment with SMTC1100, a novel small molecule utrophin upregulator, dramatically reduces the dystrophic symptoms in the mdx mouse. PLoS One. 2011;6(5):e19189.
57. Heller KN, Montgomery CL, Janssen PM, Clark KR, Mendell JR, Rodino-Klapac LR. AAV-mediated overexpression of human α7 integrin leads to histological and functional improvement in dystrophic mice. Mol Ther. 2013;21(3):520–5.
58. Amenta AR, Yilmaz A, Bogdanovich S, McKechnie BA, Abedi M, Khurana TS, Fallon JR. Biglycan recruits utrophin to the sarcolemma and counters dystrophic pathology in mdx mice. Proc Natl Acad Sci U S A. 2011;108(2):762–7.
59. Marshall JL, Kwok Y, McMorran BJ, Baum LG, Crosbie-Watson RH. The potential of sarcospan in adhesion complex replacement therapeutics for the treatment of muscular dystrophy. FEBS J. 2013;280(17):4210–29.
60. Acharyya S, Villalta SA, Bakkar N, Bupha-Intr T, Janssen PM, Carathers M, et al. Interplay of IKK/NF-KappaB signaling in macrophages and myofibers promotes muscle degeneration in Duchenne muscular dystrophy. J Clin Invest. 2007;117(4):889–901.
61. Peterson JM, Kline W, Canan BD, Ricca DJ, Kaspar B, Delfín DA, et al. Peptide-based inhibition of NF-κB rescues diaphragm muscle contractile dysfunction in a murine model of Duchenne muscular dystrophy. Mol Med. 2011;17(5–6):508–15.

62. Delfín DA, Xu Y, Peterson JM, Guttridge DC, Rafael-Fortney JA, Janssen PM. Improvement of cardiac contractile function by peptide-based inhibition of NF-κB in the utrophin/dystrophin-deficient murine model of muscular dystrophy. J Transl Med. 2011;9:68.

63. Whitehead NP, Pham C, Gervasio OL, Allen DG. N-Acetylcysteine ameliorates skeletal muscle pathophysiology in mdx mice. J Physiol. 2008;586(7):2003–14.

64. Evans NP, Call JA, Bassaganya-Riera J, Robertson JL, Grange RW. Green tea extract decreases muscle pathology and NF-kappa b immunostaining in regenerating muscle fibers of mdx mice. Clin Nutr. 2010;29(3):391–8.

65. Buyse GM, Van der Mieren G, Erb M, D'hooge J, Herijgers P, Verbeken E, et al. Long-term blinded placebo-controlled study of SNT-MC17/idebenone in the dystrophin deficient mdx mouse: cardiac protection and improved exercise performance. Eur Heart J. 2009;30(1): 116–24.

66. Buyse GM, Goemans N, van den Hauwe M, Thijs D, de Groot IJ, Schara U, et al. Idebenone as a novel, therapeutic approach for Duchenne muscular dystrophy: results from a 12 month, double-blind, randomized placebo-controlled trial. Neuromuscul Disord. 2011;21(6): 396–405.

67. Hibaoui Y, Reutenauer-Patte J, Patthey-Vuadens O, Ruegg UT, Dorchies OM. Melatonin improves muscle function of the dystrophic mdx5cv mouse, a model for Duchenne muscular dystrophy. J Pineal Res. 2011;51(2):163–71.

68. Chahbouni M, Escames G, López LC, Sevilla B, Doerrier C, Muñoz-Hoyos A, et al. Melatonin treatment counteracts the hyperoxidative status in erythrocytes of patients suffering from Duchenne muscular dystrophy. Clin Biochem. 2011;44(10–11):853–8.

69. Schertzer JD, van der Poel C, Shavlakadze T, Grounds MD, Lynch GS. Muscle-specific overexpression of IGF-I improves E-C coupling in skeletal muscle fibers from dystrophic mdx mice. Am J Physiol Cell Physiol. 2008;294(1):C161–8.

70. Secco M, Bueno C, Vieira NM, Almeida C, Pelatti M, Zucconi E, et al. Systemic delivery of human mesenchymal stromal cells combined with IGF-1 enhances muscle functional recovery in LAMA2 dy/2j dystrophic mice. Stem Cell Rev. 2013;9(1):93–109.

71. Wagner KR, Fleckenstein JL, Amato AA, Barohn RJ, Bushby K, Escolar DM, et al. A phase I/II trial of MYO-029 in adult subjects with muscular dystrophy. Ann Neurol. 2008;63(5): 561–71.

72. Rodino-Klapac LR, Janssen PM, Shontz KM, Canan B, Montgomery CL, Griffin D, et al. Micro-dystrophin and follistatin co-delivery restores muscle function in aged DMD model. Hum Mol Genet. 2013;22(24):4929–37.

73. Kainulainen H, Papaioannou KG, Silvennoinen M, Autio R, Saarela J, Oliveira BM, et al. Myostatin/activin blocking combined with exercise reconditions skeletal muscle expression profile of mdx mice. Mol Cell Endocrinol. 2015;399:131–42.

74. Cohn RD, van Erp C, Habashi JP, Soleimani AA, Klein EC, Lisi MT, et al. Angiotensin II type 1 receptor blockade attenuates TGF-beta-induced failure of muscle regeneration in multiple myopathic states. Nat Med. 2007;13(2):204–10.

75. Spurney CF, Sali A, Guerron AD, Iantorno M, Yu Q, Gordish-Dressman H, et al. Losartan decreases cardiac muscle fibrosis and improves cardiac function in dystrophin-deficient mdx mice. J Cardiovasc Pharmacol Ther. 2011;16(1):87–95.

76. Bish LT, Yarchoan M, Sleeper MM, Gazzara JA, Morine KJ, Acosta P, et al. Chronic losartan administration reduces mortality and preserves cardiac but not skeletal muscle function in dystrophic mice. PLoS One. 2011;6(6):e20856.

77. Bodanovsky A, Guttman N, Barzilai-Tutsch H, Genin O, Levy O, Pines M, Halevy O. Halofuginone improves muscle-cell survival in muscular dystrophies. Biochim Biophys Acta. 2014;1843(7):1339–47.

78. Cacchiarelli D, Martone J, Girardi E, Cesana M, Incitti T, Morlando M, et al. MicroRNAs involved in molecular circuitries relevant for the Duchenne muscular dystrophy pathogenesis are controlled by the dystrophin/nNOS pathway. Cell Metab. 2010;12(4):341–51.

79. Twayana S, Legnini I, Cesana M, Cacchiarelli D, Morlando M, Bozzoni I. Biogenesis and function of non-coding RNAs in muscle differentiation and in Duchenne muscular dystrophy. Biochem Soc Trans. 2013;41(4):844–9.

80. Bushby K, Muntoni F, Urtizberea A, Hughes R, Griggs R. Report on the 124th ENMC International Workshop. Treatment of Duchenne muscular dystrophy; defining the gold standards of management in the use of corticosteroids. 2-4 April 2004, Naarden, The Netherlands. Neuromuscul Disord. 2004;14(8–9):526–34.

81. Moxley RT, Ashwal S, Pandya S, Connolly A, Florence J, Mathews K, et al. Practice parameter: corticosteroid treatment of Duchenne dystrophy: report of the quality standards subcommittee of the American Academy of Neurology and the practice committee of the Child Neurology Society. Neurology. 2005;64(1):13–20.

82. Muntoni F, Bushby K, van Ommen G. 128th ENMC international workshop on preclinical optimization and phase I/II clinical trials using antisense oligonucleotides in Duchenne muscular dystrophy, 22–24 October 2004, Naarden, The Netherlands. Neuromuscul Disord. 2005;15(6):450–7.

83. Finder JD, Birnkrant D, Carl J, Farber HJ, Gozal D, Iannaccone ST, et al. Respiratory care of the patient with Duchenne muscular dystrophy: ATS consensus statement. Am J Respir Crit Care Med. 2004;170(4):456–65.

84. Birnkrant DJ, Bushby KM, Amin RS, Bach JR, Benditt JO, Eagle M, et al. The respiratory management of patients with Duchenne muscular dystrophy: a DMD care considerations working group specialty article. Pediatr Pulmonol. 2010;45(8):739–48.

85. American Academy of Pediatrics Section on Cardiology and Cardiac Surgery. Cardiovascular health supervision for individuals affected by Duchenne or Becker muscular dystrophy. Pediatrics. 2005;116(6):1569–73.

86. Baxter P. Treatment of the heart in Duchenne muscular dystrophy. Dev Med Child Neurol. 2006;48(3):163.

87. Mendell JR, Moxley RT, Griggs RC, Brooke MH, Fenichel GM, Miller JP, et al. Randomized, double-blind six-month trial of prednisone in Duchenne's muscular dystrophy. N Engl J Med. 1989;320(24):1592–7.

88. Griggs RC, Moxley RT, Mendell JR, Fenichel GM, Brooke MH, Pestronk A, Miller JP. Prednisone in Duchenne dystrophy. A randomized, controlled trial defining the time course and dose response. Clinical Investigation of Duchenne Dystrophy Group. Arch Neurol. 1991;48(4):383–8.

89. Biggar WD, Gingras M, Fehlings DL, Harris VA, Steele CA. Deflazacort treatment of Duchenne muscular dystrophy. J Pediatr. 2001;138(1):45–50.

90. Schara U, Mortier J, Mortier W. Long-term steroid therapy in Duchenne muscular dystrophy-positive results versus side effects. J Clin Neuromuscul Dis. 2001;2(4):179–83.

91. Kinali M, Main M, Eliahoo J, Messina S, Knight RK, Lehovsky J, et al. Predictive factors for the development of scoliosis in Duchenne muscular dystrophy. Eur J Paediatr Neurol. 2007;11(3):160–6.

92. Markham LW, Kinnett K, Wong BL, Woodrow Benson D, Cripe LH. Corticosteroid treatment retards development of ventricular dysfunction in Duchenne muscular dystrophy. Neuromuscul Disord. 2008;18(5):365–70.

93. Henricson EK, Abresch RT, Cnaan A, Hu F, Duong T, Arrieta A, et al. The cooperative international neuromuscular research group Duchenne natural history study: glucocorticoid treatment preserves clinically meaningful functional milestones and reduces rate of disease progression as measured by manual muscle testing and other commonly used clinical trial outcome measures. Muscle Nerve. 2013;48(1):55–67.

94. McAdam LC, Mayo AL, Alman BA, Biggar WD. The Canadian experience with long-term deflazacort treatment in Duchenne muscular dystrophy. Acta Myol. 2012;31(1):16–20.

95. Morgenroth VH, Hache LP, Clemens PR. Insights into bone health in Duchenne muscular dystrophy. Bonekey Rep. 2012;1:9.

96. Sbrocchi AM, Rauch F, Jacob P, McCormick A, McMillan HJ, Matzinger MA, Ward LM. The use of intravenous bisphosphonate therapy to treat vertebral fractures due to osteoporosis among boys with Duchenne muscular dystrophy. Osteoporos Int. 2012;23(11):2703–11.

97. Houston C, Mathews K, Shibli-Rahhal A. Bone density and alendronate effects in Duchenne muscular dystrophy patients. Muscle Nerve. 2014;49(4):506–11.

98. Judge DP, Kass DA, Thompson WR, Wagner KR. Pathophysiology and therapy of cardiac dysfunction in Duchenne muscular dystrophy. Am J Cardiovasc Drugs. 2011;11(5):287–94.
99. Passamano L, Taglia A, Palladino A, Viggiano E, D'Ambrosio P, Scutifero M, et al. Improvement of survival in Duchenne muscular dystrophy: retrospective analysis of 835 patients. Acta Myol. 2012;31(2):121–5.
100. Nigro G, Comi LI, Politano L, Bain RJ. The incidence and evolution of cardiomyopathy in Duchenne muscular dystrophy. Int J Cardiol. 1990;26(3):271–7.
101. Spurney CF. Cardiomyopathy of Duchenne muscular dystrophy: current understanding and future directions. Muscle Nerve. 2011;44(1):8–19.
102. Bilchick KC, Salerno M, Plitt D, Dori Y, Crawford TO, Drachman D, Thompson WR. Prevalence and distribution of regional scar in dysfunctional myocardial segments in Duchenne muscular dystrophy. J Cardiovasc Magn Reson. 2011;13:20.
103. Romfh A, McNally EM. Cardiac assessment in Duchenne and Becker muscular dystrophies. Curr Heart Fail Rep. 2010;7:212–8.
104. Bach JR, Martinez D. Duchenne muscular dystrophy: continuous noninvasive ventilatory support prolongs survival. Respir Care. 2011;56(6):744–50.
105. McKim DA, Katz SL, Barrowman N, Ni A, LeBlanc C. Lung volume recruitment slows pulmonary function decline in Duchenne muscular dystrophy. Arch Phys Med Rehabil. 2012;93(7):1117–22.
106. Bach JR, Sinquee DM, Saporito LR, Botticello AL. Efficacy of mechanical insufflation-exsufflation in extubating unweanable subjects with restrictive pulmonary disorders. Respir Care. 2014.
107. Davidson ZE, Truby H. A review of nutrition in Duchenne muscular dystrophy. J Hum Nutr Diet. 2009;22(5):383–93.
108. Nereo NE, Fee RJ, Hinton VJ. Parental stress in mothers of boys with Duchenne muscular dystrophy. J Pediatr Psychol. 2003;28(7):473–84.
109. Pangalila RF, van den Bos GA, Stam HJ, van Exel NJ, Brouwer WB, Roebroeck ME. Subjective caregiver burden of parents of adults with Duchenne muscular dystrophy. Disabil Rehabil. 2012;34(12):988–96.
110. Mah JK, Thannhauser JE, Kolski H, Dewey D. Parental stress and quality of life in children with neuromuscular disease. Pediatr Neurol. 2008;39(2):102–7.
111. Mah JK, Thannhauser JE, MacNeil DA, Dewey D. Being the lifeline: the parent experience of caring for a child with neuromuscular disease on home mechanical ventilation. Neuromuscul Disord. 2008;18(12):983–8.
112. Samson A, Tomiak E, Dimillo J, Lavigne R, Miles S, Choquette M, et al. The lived experience of hope among parents of a child with Duchenne muscular dystrophy: perceiving the human being beyond the illness. Chronic Illn. 2009;5(2):103–14.

# Chapter 5
# An Overview of the Other Muscular Dystrophies: Underlying Genetic and Molecular Mechanisms

Jean K. Mah

## Introduction

Muscular dystrophies (MDs) refer to a heterogeneous group of disorders associated with on going muscle degeneration and regeneration, leading to progressive weakness. They can be transmitted as autosomal dominant, autosomal recessive, or X-linked pattern of inheritance; sporadic cases may also arise as a result of de novo mutation, in the absence of any family history of affected individuals. The distribution of weakness in MDs includes a limb-girdle pattern, with shoulder and hip girdle muscle involvement; a humeroperoneal pattern, with predominantly triceps, biceps, and peroneal muscles weakness; or a distal pattern, with distal weakness in the legs and arms [1]. Examples of MDs include congenital muscular dystrophy (CMD), myotonic dystrophy (DM), limb girdle muscular dystrophy (LGMD), Emery–Dreifuss muscular dystrophy (EDMD), oculopharyngeal muscular dystrophy (OPMD), facioscapulohumeral muscular dystrophy (FSHD), Duchenne muscular dystrophy (DMD), and Becker muscular dystrophy (BMD). According to Emery, the prevalence of MDs ranged from 1.3 to 96.2 per million, with DMD being most prevalent among boys during childhood, and myotonic dystrophy as one of the most common forms of MDs worldwide [2].

Traditionally, the classification of MDs is based on a combination of clinical and pathological criteria, including the age of onset and distribution of muscle weakness, the extent of disease progression, associated symptoms, systemic features, family history, serum creatine kinase, muscle histology, as well as electromyography and nerve conduction studies (EMG/NCS). Increasingly, the diagnosis of MDs requires

J.K. Mah, M.D., M.Sc. (✉)
Department of Pediatrics and Clinical Neurosciences, University of Calgary, Alberta
Children's Hospital, 2888 Shaganappi Trail NW, Calgary, AB, Canada, T3B 6A8
e-mail: jean.mah@albertahealthservices.ca

© Springer International Publishing Switzerland 2015
R.A. Huml (ed.), *Muscular Dystrophy*, DOI 10.1007/978-3-319-17362-7_5

genetic confirmation, as there can be considerable variations and overlaps in the clinical phenotypes [3]. The differential diagnosis of MDs includes other inherited and acquired causes of muscle weakness such as inflammatory myopathies, congenital or metabolic myopathies, non-dystrophic myotonias, muscle channelopathies, motor neuron diseases, neuropathies, and neuromuscular junction transmission defects; a careful neurological examination plus appropriate ancillary tests should be performed to exclude these disorders [4]. This chapter aims to provide an overview of the myotonic dystrophies, LGMDs, and congenital muscular dystrophies. Duchenne and Becker muscular dystrophy as well as facioscapulohumeral dystrophy are discussed in other chapters.

# Myotonic Dystrophies

Myotonic dystrophies are autosomal dominant disorders associated with myotonia, progressive muscular weakness, as well as extramuscular manifestations such as cardiac arrhythmia, cataracts, endocrine dysfunction, and variable degrees of central nervous system involvement. These diseases are classified as type 1 or type 2 myotonic dystrophy, based on clinical features as well as molecular genetic diagnosis. Type 1 myotonic dystrophy is due to an abnormal expansion of trinucleotide (CTG) repeats located in the 3′-untranslated region of the dystrophia myotonica protein kinase gene, located on chromosome 19q13.3 [5, 6]. Type 2 myotonic dystrophy is caused by an expansion of tetranucleotide (CCTG) repeats in intron 1 of the zinc finger protein 9 (ZNF9) gene, located on chromosome 3q21.3 [7, 8]; it is also known as proximal myotonic myopathy (PROMM) [9] or proximal myotonic dystrophy (PDM) [10]. The expanded repeats in both types of myotonic dystrophies are associated with intranuclear accumulations of ribonucleic acid (RNA) inclusions, resulting in abnormal interactions with RNA-binding proteins and misregulation of developmentally programmed alternative splicing [11, 12]. The altered distribution of muscleblind-like 1 and CUG-binding proteins adversely affects transcription, translation, and cell signaling functions [13, 14]. Furthermore, nuclear sequestration of muscleblind-like proteins inhibits myoblast differentiation and impairs muscle regeneration [15, 16]. Moreover, it has been shown that the highly regulated pathways of miRNA are altered in skeletal muscle and heart tissues, thus potentially contributing to disease pathogenesis [17, 18].

## *Type 1 Myotonic Dystrophy*

Type 1 myotonic dystrophy (DM1) is one of the most common forms of MD in adulthood, with an estimated prevalence of 1 in 8,000 [19]. It is subdivided into several clinical phenotypes depending on the age of presentation, including the congenital, early childhood, adult, and late onset forms. Normal alleles range from 5 to 37 CTG repeats. An abnormal increase in CTG beyond 50 repeats is unstable and may result in further expansion in the germline, leading to genetic anticipation with more severe weakness and earlier onset of disease in successive generations among affected families [20, 21]. In the severe congenital form of myotonic dystrophy type 1, 1,000 or more CTG repeats may be demonstrated, while 50–1,000 repeats are seen in the later onset form of the disease [22–25].

**Congenital Myotonic Dystrophy**

Infants with this severe form of type 1 myotonic dystrophy are overtly symptomatic at birth [26]. The mother is the affected parent in most cases, and polyhydramnios is commonly reported during the pregnancy because of inadequate fetal swallowing of amniotic fluid [27, 28]. Common neonatal manifestations include joint contractures, ranging from equinovarus deformities of the feet to arthrogryposis multiplex congenita, hypotonia, and generalized weakness [29]. The characteristic facies with facial diplegia, inverted V-shaped upper lip, temporalis wasting, small chin, and high-arched palate may be the first clues to the diagnosis [30]. Dysphagia is common; infants may require gavage feeding and/or subsequent gastrostomy placement due to persistence of oral motor dysfunction during childhood [31, 32]. Respiratory insufficiency also affects a significant proportion of neonates; infants with congenital myotonic dystrophy may require supplementary oxygen, positive airway pressure by nasal prongs or masks, or in some cases tracheostomy and long-term mechanical ventilation. Neonates requiring ventilatory support for more than 30 days, in particular, had increased mortality during the first year, according to a retrospective review [33]. Survivors may have chronic complications related to poor GI motility, myotonia, cardiac arrhythmias, impaired visual function, and cataracts [34]. Learning disabilities and mental retardation are also common complications in congenital DM1 [35, 36]; neuroimaging studies may show ventriculomegaly and abnormal cerebral white matter changes [37, 38]. Furthermore, affected children and adolescents are at increased risk for neuropsychiatric co-morbidities such as autistic spectrum conditions or attention deficit disorder [39, 40]. Even though their muscle tone and strength may improve beyond the neonatal period, children with congenital myotonic dystrophy generally remain developmentally delayed. On going issues including cognitive impairment, behavioral challenges, and learning disability will require multidisciplinary support.

**Childhood Onset Myotonic Dystrophy**

Childhood onset type 1 myotonic dystrophy can be transmitted from either parent. These children have similar symptoms to those with the congenital form of the disease, but these are generally less severe and present at a later age. Cognitive deficits and learning abnormalities may occasionally be the presenting complaints [41].

**Adult Onset Myotonic Dystrophy**

Patients with adult onset type 1 myotonic dystrophy are generally recognized by their clinical appearance with ptosis, facial weakness, temporalis muscle wasting, myotonia, as well as a combination of proximal and distal muscle weakness. Difficulty with muscle relaxation can result in problems with chewing, swallowing, and talking due to involvement of the bulbar, tongue, or facial muscles, in addition to the positive grip and percussion myotonia. Posterior subcapsular cataracts, obstructive sleep apnea, irritable bowel syndrome, and cardiac conduction defects are common; the latter is a significant contributor to morbidity and mortality in myotonic dystrophy [42, 43]. Endocrine dysfunction may develop, leading to testicular atrophy, type 2 diabetes mellitus, and hypothyroidism. Intellectual impairment, if present, is generally milder than with the childhood onset subtypes. Personality profiles including obsessive-compulsive, avoidant, and passive-aggressive traits have also been described [44, 45].

**Late-Onset Myotonic Dystrophy Type 1**

Individuals with mild expansion of CTG repeats may remain largely asymptomatic, apart from early onset cataracts. Myotonia may also be detected on clinical assessment [19].

## Type 2 Myotonic Dystrophy (DM2)

In myotonic dystrophy type 2, two clinical phenotypes have been described: PROMM and PDM [9, 10, 46]. Both conditions typically affect adults and are linked to myotonia, early-onset cataracts, and proximal muscle weakness. In addition to the aforementioned genetic differences, there are a number of unique features in myotonic dystrophy type 2. In contrast to myotonic dystrophy type 1, type 2 myotonic dystrophy has not been associated with a congenital form of disease, and cognitive or behavioral problems are rare [47, 48]. If present, cognitive impairment in type 2 myotonic dystrophy is generally mild [47, 49]. Furthermore, muscle pain can be a severe and disabling problem for individuals with type 2 myotonic dystrophy, but not usually for those with type 1 disease [19]. In particular, muscle stiffness and pain are more common in PROMM [10, 50, 51]. Both PROMM and PDM can be associated with cardiac conduction defects; sudden death and severe cardiac arrhythmias have been described in small numbers of patients [51, 52]. Endocrine dysfunction may also occur and can worsen over time [53, 54].

## Diagnostic Workup

The history and neurology examination is an important first step in the diagnostic approach. A detailed family history including examination of the parents (particularly of the mother in infants with congenital myotonic dystrophy) is essential. The serum creatine kinase is usually mildly elevated. Electromyography studies may reveal electrical myotonia and a myopathic pattern, but such findings may be absent or non-specific in early childhood. The single most important confirmatory diagnostic test is the molecular genetic marker for myotonic dystrophy. Muscle biopsy is now rarely indicated unless genetic testing is equivocal or not available. Roentgenograms of the chest and abdomen can help determine the status of diaphragmatic and gastrointestinal functions. A swallow study may also be indicated for infants with feeding difficulties; similarly, close respiratory monitoring including pulmonary function test, overnight pulse oximetry, and formal sleep studies are required to detect early respiratory insufficiency [55]. An echocardiography should also be performed periodically for all individuals with myotonic dystrophy, even if clinically asymptomatic [56]. Serial electrocardiograms (ECG) are also required on a regular basis to monitor for cardiac arrhythmia. The eyes should be examined with a slit-lamp for early onset cataracts; standard direct ophthalmoscopy may not be adequate. Endocrine monitoring including serum cortisol, thyroid function, insulin, and blood glucose should be performed periodically. Prenatal diagnosis is available from chorionic villus samples and cultured amniocytes, from which DNA analysis can be performed during the first half of gestation at 8–20 weeks. Fetal cord blood may be obtained in older fetuses and genetic studies performed on leukocytes. Additional guidelines for molecular approaches to the myotonic dystrophies are available [57–59].

## Management

In general, the management of the myotonic dystrophies remains largely supportive. Bracing may help with distal muscle weakness such as foot drop, and devices such as scooters or wheelchairs can help conserve energy and/or improve mobility. In specific circumstances, anti-myotonic agents may be helpful, especially if muscle stiffness is frequent and persistent or if pain is prominent [60].

## Congenital Muscular Dystrophy

CMD refers a heterogeneous group of early onset MDs, with an estimated prevalence ranging from 0.68 to 2.5 per 100,000 [61–64]. Affected children are usually symptomatic at birth or before their first six months of life. The salient features include hypotonia, muscle weakness, reduced deep tendon reflexes, with or without joint contractures. Feeding and respiratory insufficiency are common due to associated bulbar and respiratory muscle involvement. Additional features may include microcephaly, eye anomalies, cerebral malformation, joint laxity, muscle atrophy or hypertrophy, adducted thumbs, and skin changes. Based on the underlying pathophysiology, the congenital muscular dystrophies can be further subdivided into disorders involving (a) the basal lamina or extracellular matrix proteins; (b) α dystroglycanopathy; (c) sarcoplasmic reticulum calcium release channel; (d) endoplasmic reticulum proteins; (e) nuclear envelope proteins, (f) mitochondrial membrane proteins; and (g) other unspecified dystrophies [65].

The differential diagnosis of CMD includes congenital myopathies, congenital myasthenic syndromes, early onset spinal muscular atrophy, congenital neuropathies, as well as other metabolic and genetic conditions. The approaches to the differential diagnosis include electromyography and nerve conduction studies to exclude neurogenic involvement or neuromuscular junction transmission disorders, selective biochemical or genetic testing, as well neuroimaging studies and muscle biopsy. As seen with other dystrophies, the muscle biopsy in CMD usually demonstrates dystrophic changes with degeneration, necrosis, and regeneration, plus variable degrees of fibrosis and fatty replacement. Serum creatine kinase can range from normal to significantly elevated. Electromyography may reveal an associated peripheral neuropathy, in addition to myopathic changes in certain subtypes of CMD. Furthermore, brain MRI may reveal central nervous system malformations as well as white matter changes.

# Diagnostic Aspects of Specific Subtypes

## *Laminin Alpha 2-Related or Merosin-Deficient CMD*

Mutations in the LAMA2 gene located on Ch 6q22-23 result in merosin-deficient CMD. The gene encodes the alpha 2 heavy chain of the laminin 211 isoform, which is also known as merosin [66, 67]. Patients with complete merosin deficiency present at birth with severe hypotonia, proximal more than distal muscle weakness, and multiple joint contractures. Respiratory insufficiency and feeding difficulties are common. Affected children with complete deficiency seldom achieve independent ambulation. Brain MRI may show hyperintense T2-weighted and fluid attenuated inversion recovery (FLAIR) changes affecting the subcortical white matter; similarly, nerve conduction study may reveal a demyelinating polyneuropathy as merosin is also expressed in central and peripheral myelin. Cognition is generally normal. A small minority of children may have additional brain anomalies including occipital cortical dysplasia, subcortical band heterotopia, and cerebellar hypoplasia [68]; approximately 30% of children with merosin-deficient CMD may have associated seizure disorders.

## *Alpha-Dystroglycan-Related Dystrophies*

Alpha-dystroglycan is an integral sarcolemmal membrane protein. Defects in glycosylation of alpha-dystroglycan result in a number of disorders including CMD. The spectrum of involvement may include prenatal onset weakness precluding ambulation to a variable degree of LGMDs. There are currently 13 genes directly or putatively involved in the glycosylation pathway, including POMT1, POMT2, POMGnT1, FKRP, Fukutin, LARGE, ISPD, GTDC2, B3GALNT2, B3GNT1, TMEM5, GMPPB, SGK196 [69, 70]. Mutation in dystroglycan (DAG1) that specifically interferes with its glycosylation can also lead to alpha-dystroglycan-related dystrophies [71]. Additional mutations in the dolichyl-phosphate mannosyltransferase subunit genes of DPM1, DPM2, and DPM3 can cause an overlapping of syndromes of MD with under-glycosylated alpha-dystroglycan [72–74]. A range of central nervous system involvement including type II lissencephaly, polymicrogyria, pachygyria, brainstem, or cerebellar dysplasia may be present on brain MRI studies. Variable degrees of cognitive impairment including severe mental retardation and learning disability have also been observed. In addition, mutations involving the FKRP and FKTN genes are more likely to be associated with dilated cardiomyopathy.

## *Collagen VI-Related Dystrophies*

Collagen VI deficiency results in a spectrum of disorders ranging from severe CMD to a milder form of Bethlem myopathy [75, 76]. It is related to mutation of one of three collagen VI alpha genes, located on Ch 2q (A3) or 21q22 (A1 & A2). The disease can be inherited in an autosomal recessive or dominant fashion. Clinical features of collagen VI-related dystrophies or Ullrich CMD include hypotonia, proximal more than distal weakness, marked distal joint hyperlaxity, skin changes, and progressive contractures from birth. Respiratory and feeding problems are common, leading to failure to thrive and nocturnal hypoventilation [77, 78]. Cognition is normal and may be advanced for age. CK can be normal or minimally elevated. Affected individuals may lose independent ambulation during childhood [79]. Characteristic skin findings are diagnostically helpful and include a tendency for keloid or atrophic scar formation, striae, and hyperkeratosis pilaris [80]. Serum creatine kinase is normal or mildly elevated.

## *SEPN1-Related Myopathy*

SEPN1-related myopathies are autosomal recessive disorders caused by mutations of the SEPN1 gene on 1p3. This encodes selenoprotein N (SelN), an endoplasmic reticulum protein that plays an essential role in protecting human cells against oxidative stress [81, 82]. Mutations of SEPN1 can result in either a congenital myopathy or a more severe CMD phenotype. The key features include early onset weakness, particular involving the axial muscle groups, including neck flexor and sometimes extensor weakness, leading to a "dropped head" phenotype [83, 84]. In contrast, strength in the extremities is generally preserved until later in life. Other clinical features include distal hyperlaxity, facial weakness, and relative atrophy of the inner thigh muscles; nocturnal hypoventilation may be evident after the first decade of life due to restrictive pulmonary function [85]. Progression is slow, with reduced independent mobility after the fourth decade of life. Serum creatine kinase is normal or mildly elevated.

## RYR1-Related Myopathy

Autosomal recessive mutations in the RYR1 gene can result in a distinct CMD-like presentation (RYR1-CMD), in addition to the congenital myopathy phenotype. The gene encodes for the sarcoplasmic reticulum calcium release channel. It is allelic to other recessive RYR1-related myopathies that include centronuclear, central core, multi-minicore, congenital fiber type disproportion, as well as other non-specific histological presentations [86, 87]. Affected children with RYR1-CMD may present with a histological and clinical picture suggestive of CMD. Unlike RYR1-related congenital myopathy, RYR1-CMD may lack the features of core formation on muscle biopsy [65].

## Lamin A/C-Related CMD

Mutations in the lamin A/C (LMNA) gene result in a spectrum of genetic disorders in humans, including CMD and LGMDs [88, 89]. Lamin A/C is part of the nuclear membrane proteins. In LMNA-CMD, weakness becomes evident in infancy; severe axial and neck muscle involvement may result in a dropped head syndrome [90, 91] due to prominent neck extensor weakness. In addition, there is often pronounced lumbar hyperlordosis at a very early age, with arm and hand weakness as well as peroneal predominant weakness, as seen with an early axial–scapulo–peroneal pattern of involvement. Progressive weakness may lead to motor developmental regression early in life, with loss of independent ambulation as well as other gross motor milestones before age 3. Feeding, cardiac, and respiratory complications are common, leading to nocturnal hypoventilation before the end of the first decade of life [92]. Cognition is normal. Serum creatine kinase levels can be mildly to moderately elevated. The cardiac manifestation in lamin A/C-related CMD may take the form of an initially atrial arrhythmogenic cardiomyopathy with conduction block; subsequent development of ventricular tachyarrhythmias requires the use of an automatic implantable cardioverter defibrillator (AICD).

## *Mutations in Metabolic (Mitochondrial Membrane Protein) Pathway Genes*

Several genetic causes for CMD like presentations have been described recently and involve mutations in genes involved in the metabolic pathways, including choline kinase B in 22q13. The gene is involved in phosphatidylcholine biosynthesis; mutations result in a congenital onset MD. Muscle biopsy reveals abnormally large mitochondria on oxidative stains and ultrastructure, in addition to dystrophic changes [93]. The constellation of clinical signs together with the biopsy findings of mitochondria depleted in center of muscle fibers, accumulated and enlarged at the periphery, is diagnostic of CHKB-related CMD. Dilated cardiomyopathy may develop over time. Affected patients in addition show cognitive impairment but normal brain MRI findings. Skin changes may include acanthosis nigricans and ichthyosis [65].

## *Other Congenital Muscular Dystrophies*

Integrin α7 (*ITGA7*) is a transmembrane laminin receptor, located on chromosome 12q13. Deficiency of integrin α7 is a rare cause of CMD. Similarly, integrin α9 deficiency (*ITGA9*) related to mutations on 3p23-21 has also been described from French Canadian families. The clinical feature is similar to Ullrich CMD but is generally less severe [65].

Management of congenital muscular dystrophies includes genetic counseling for family and relatives, physical therapy, range of motion stretching exercises, and supportive strategies for mobility, respiratory, and feeding issues. Use of mechanical assistive devices as well as surgery for scoliosis and gastrostomy tube placement may be required. Regular cardiac respiratory monitoring is essential. The overall life expectancy in CMD is presently unknown. Premature death may result from respiratory and cardiac complications. In one series of merosin-deficient CMD, the mortality rate was approximately 20% (4 out of 22 patients) during childhood, with death occurring between five and ten years of age [94].

## Limb-Girdle Muscular Dystrophy

LGMD refers to a heterogeneous group of autosomal muscular dystrophies with progressive weakness affecting predominantly the hip and shoulder girdles. The facial and distal muscles are generally spared early on in the disease. Historically, the MDs are classified as either type 1 (dominant) or type 2 (recessive) depending on the mode of inheritance. As well, the disorders are labeled consecutively by the alphabet according to when the individual genes were identified. The main classes of proteins involved in these conditions are extracellular matrix and external membrane proteins, enzymes or proteins with putative enzymatic function, sarcolemma-associated proteins, nuclear membrane proteins, sarcomeric proteins, and others [1]. The diagnostic approach for LGMD is often challenging because of significant disease heterogeneity.

In addition to the distribution of weakness, ethnicity, and family history, clues to the diagnosis of LGMD include age of onset of symptoms, rate of disease progression, presence of associated signs such as contracture, rigidity, rippling muscle, muscle hypertrophy or atrophy, as well as systemic involvement including cardiac, pulmonary, and skin complications [1]. By definition, the term "limb-girdle muscular dystrophy" usually excludes other defined types of MDs such as Duchenne and Becker MD, myotonic dystrophies, and FSHD [4]. An understanding regarding the epidemiology of various MDs is also helpful. Among LGMD, the recessive forms are generally more prevalent than the dominant variants in certain regions, including LGMD 2A in southern Europe, and LGMD 2I, followed by LGMD 2B in northern Europe. Substantial overlaps exist, as mutations in different proteins that share similar cellular functions can result in nearly identical clinical phenotypes. Conversely, allelic disorders can give rise to divergent diseases, as may be seen in lamin A/C (LMNA) gene mutations resulting in EDMD, LGMD 1B, as well as axonal Charcot-Marie-Tooth disease and several other phenotypes with no muscle involvement [1].

Accordingly to Nigro and Savarese [95], there are currently eight subtypes of autosomal-dominant (type 1) LGMD. The genes and respective locus involved include myotilin, on 5q31.2 (1A); lamin A/C, on 1q22 (1B); caveolin 3, on 3q25.3; DNAJ/Hsp40 homolog subfamily B member 6, on 7q36 (1D); desmin, on 2q35 (1E); transportin 3, on 7q32 (1F); heterogeneous nuclear ribonucleoprotein D-like protein, on 4q21 (1G); and an un-named gene, on 3p23-p25 (1H). Similarly, there are 23 subtypes of autosomal recessive (type 2) LGMD. The genes and respective locus include calpain 3, on 15q15 (2A); dysferlin, on 2q13.2 (2B); $\gamma$-sarcoglycan, on 13q12 (2C); $\alpha$-sarcoglycan, on 17q21.33 (2D); $\beta$-sarcoglycan, on 4q12 (2E); $\delta$-sarcoglycan, on 5q33 (2F); telethonin, on 17q12 (2G); tripartite motif containing 32, on 9q33.1 (2H); fukutin-related protein, on 19q13.3 (2I); titin, on 2q24.3 (2J); protein-$O$-mannosyl transferase 1, on 9q34.1 (2K); anoctamin 5, on 11p13-p12 (2L); fukutin, on 9q31 (2M); protein-$O$-mannosyl transferase 2, on 14q24 (2N); protein-O-linked mannose beta 1,2-$N$-acetylglucosaminyl transferase, on 1p34.1 (2O); dystroglycan, on 3p21 (2P); plectin, on 8q24 (2Q); desmin, on 2q35 (2R); transport protein particle complex 11, on 4q35 (2S); GDP-mannose pyrophosphorylase B, on 3p21 (2T); isoprenoid synthase domain containing, on 7p21 (2U); alpha-1, 4-glucosidase, on 17q25.3 (2V); and lim and senescent cell antigen-like domains 2, on 2q14 (2W) [95].

The differential diagnosis of LGMD is broad; it includes other MDs such as congenital muscular dystrophies, myotonic dystrophy, FSHD, and EDMD, as well as congenital myopathies, myofibrillar myopathies, distal myopathies, metabolic myopathy (such as Pompe or lipid storage disease), channelopathies, inflammatory myopathies, neurogenic disorders, and neuromuscular junction transmission disorders.

## Example 1: LGMD 2D, α-Sarcoglycanopathy with a Duchenne-Like Phenotype

A seven-year-old girl presented with a three-year history of progressive difficulty walking and high serum CK. Her exam was noted for proximal muscle weakness, mild calf hypertrophy, scapular winging, and Achilles tendon contractures. She had a positive Gowers sign, and she walked with a waddling gait with increased lumbar lordosis. Her muscle biopsy showed dystrophic changes with pronounced reduction of α-sarcoglycan and mildly reduced dystrophin on immunostaining. Subsequent genetic analysis confirmed that the primary abnormality is due to mutation of α-sarcoglycan.

## Example 2: LGMD 2I, FKRP Dystroglycanopathies

A 12-year-old boy presented with a 5-year history of difficulty with running and high serum CK. His older sister was previously diagnosed with a type of LGMD based on muscle biopsy showing dystrophic features. His exam was noted for proximal hip and shoulder girdle weakness, with calf hypertrophy, and mild bilateral heel cord contractures. Molecular genetic testing for dystrophinopathy was negative. Mutations in the fukutin-related protein gene FKRP (19q13.3) were found by molecular genetic testing, thus confirming the diagnosis of limb-girdle muscular dystrophy type 2I (LGMD2I).

## Example 3: LGMD 2A, Calpainopathy

A 24-year-old woman presented with insidious onset of muscle weakness and difficulty climbing stairs. Her serum CK was moderately elevated. Her exam revealed proximal more than distal muscle weakness; the weakest muscles involved the hip adductors and extensors, with mild contractures in her heel cords and hamstring. Molecular genetic testing confirmed a mutation of calpain 3, which belongs to a family of calcium-activated neutral proteases. Calpain 3 interacts with several proteins including dysferlin and titin that are crucial for muscle function. It is one of the most common forms of autosomal recessive LGMD, with a reported frequency ranging from 9 to 40% in published series [1].

## Example 4: LGMD 1B, Laminopathy

An 18-year-old man presented with a long-standing history of gross motor developmental delay and elevated CK. His father had similar history of muscle weakness and died prematurely due to cardiac arrest. His exam limb girdle distribution of muscle weakness, with mild contractures and reduced subcutaneous fat in his extremities. Cardiac work revealed prolonged QTc interval with atrial tachyarrhythmia. He was subsequently confirmed to have LGMD 1B due to a mutation in the LMNA gene.

## *Example 5:* **LGMD 2B,** *Dysferlinopathy*

A 16-year-old athletic teenager presented with a 2-year history of exercise-induced myalgia. He was found to have moderately elevated serum CK. His examination was normal apart from mild proximal muscle weakness. Muscle biopsy revealed a mildly dystrophic pattern with reduced immunostaining for dysferlin. Subsequent genetic testing confirmed a diagnosis of LGMD2B. LGMD2B is a relatively mild disease with a predominantly proximal slowly progressive involvement of the pelvic and shoulder girdles presenting in the late second or third decade of life. It is linked to Ch2p12-14 [96]. Individuals are often normal or even athletic in their early years. Mutation in the dysferin gene is associated with several phenotypes, including LGMD 2B, Miyoshi myopathy, and distal anterior compartment myopathy. Miyoshi myopathy presents with early involvement of the posterior compartment of the lower extremities, with inability to stand on the toes [97]. Another allelic disorder results in a distal anterior compartment myopathy, with inability to stand on heels due to rapidly progressive weakness of the anterior tibial muscles [98].

## **Diagnosis and Management of LGMD**

Similar to other MDs, the approach to LGMD requires a detailed history, a thorough physical examination, and serum creatine kinase level. Other genetic and acquired causes of proximal muscular weakness should be excluded. The diagnosis may be confirmed by molecular genetic testing, muscle biopsy, or a combination of both. Muscle biopsy will typically reveal the characteristic dystrophic features; further immunostaining may demonstrate the presence or absence of specific muscle proteins such as dystrophin, dysferlin, sarcoglycans, emerin, collagen VI, merosin, and glycosylated alpha-dystroglycan. Women should also be offered appropriate testing to exclude manifesting carrier of dystrophinopathy as a potential cause for their MD. The future of molecular testing may shift away from targeted genetic analysis toward whole genome or exome sequencing that will allow rapid and cost-efficient means of confirming the diagnosis. General treatment principles include offering genetic counseling for affected individuals and families, connecting them with patient organization and disease registries, providing rehabilitation through multidisciplinary clinics to maximize function, supporting education, career, social, and financial needs, screening and treating the associated complications, and evaluating new treatment options for specific diseases when available.

# References

1. Mercuri E, Muntoni F. Muscular dystrophies. Lancet. 2013;381:845–60.
2. Emery AE. Population frequencies of inherited neuromuscular diseases—a world survey. Neuromuscul Disord. 1991;1:19–29.
3. Arnold WD, Flanigan KM. A practical approach to molecular diagnostic testing in neuromuscular diseases. Phys Med Rehabil Clin N Am. 2012;23:589–608.
4. Narayanaswami P, Weiss M, Selcen D, David W, Raynor E, Carter G, et al. Evidence-based guideline summary: diagnosis and treatment of limb-girdle and distal dystrophies: report of the guideline development subcommittee of the American Academy of Neurology and the practice issues review panel of the American Association of Neuromuscular & Electrodiagnostic Medicine. Neurology. 2014;83:1453–63.
5. Brook JD, McCurrach ME, Harley HG, et al. Molecular basis of myotonic dystrophy: expansion of a trinucleotide (CTG) repeat at the 3′ end of a transcript encoding a protein kinase family member. Cell. 1992;68:799–808.
6. Fu YH, Pizzuti A, Fenwick Jr RG, et al. An unstable triplet repeat in a gene related to myotonic muscular dystrophy. Science. 1992;255:1256–8.
7. Ranum LP, Rasmussen PF, Benzow KA, Koob MD, Day JW. Genetic mapping of a second myotonic dystrophy locus. Nat Genet. 1998;19:196–8.
8. Liquori CL, Ricker K, Moseley ML, Jacobsen JF, Kress W, Naylor SL, et al. Myotonic dystrophy type 2 caused by a CCTG expansion in intron 1 of ZNF9. Science. 2001;293:864–7.
9. Ricker K, Koch MC, Lehmann-Horn F, Pongratz D, Otto M, Heine R, Moxley RT. Proximal myotonic myopathy: a new dominant disorder with myotonia, muscle weakness, and cataracts. Neurology. 1994;44:1448–52.
10. Udd B, Krahe R, Wallgren-Pettersson C, Falck B, Kalimo H. Proximal myotonic dystrophy—a family with autosomal dominant muscular dystrophy, cataracts, hearing loss and hypogonadism: heterogeneity of proximal myotonic syndromes? Neuromuscul Disord. 1997;7:217–28.
11. Lin X, Miller JW, Mankodi A, et al. Failure of MBNL1-dependent post-natal splicing transitions in myotonic dystrophy. Hum Mol Genet. 2006;15:2087–97.
12. Wojciechowska M, Krzyzosiak WJ. Cellular toxicity of expanded RNA repeats: focus on RNA foci. Hum Mol Genet. 2011;20:3811–21.
13. Pascual M, Vincente M, Monferrer L, Artero R. The muscleblind family of proteins: an emerging class of regulators of developmentally programmed alternative splicing. Differentiation. 2006;74:65–80.
14. Barreau C, Paillard L, Méreau A, Osborne HB. Mammalian CELF/bruno-like RNA-binding proteins: molecular characteristics and biological functions. Biochimie. 2006;88:515–25.
15. Amack JD, Mahadevan MS. Myogenic defects in myotonic dystrophy. Dev Biol. 2004;265:294–301.
16. Cardani R, Mancinelli E, Rotondo G, Sansone V, Meola G. Muscleblind-like protein 1 nuclear sequestration is a molecular pathology marker of DM1 and DM2. Eur J Histochem. 2006;50:177–82.
17. Perbellini R, Greco S, Sarra-Ferraris G, Cardani R, Capogrossi MC, Meola G, Martelli F. Dysregulation and cellular mislocalization of specific miRNAs in myotonic dystrophy type 1. Neuromuscul Disord. 2011;21:81–8.
18. Greco S, Perfetti A, Fasanaro P, Cardani R, Capogrossi MC, Meola G, Martelli F. Deregulated microRNAs in myotonic dystrophy type 2. PLoS One. 2012;7:e39732.
19. Meola G. Clinical aspects, molecular pathomechanisms and management of myotonic dystrophies. Acta Myol. 2013;32:154–65.
20. Abbruzzese C, Costanzi Porrini S, Mariani B, et al. Instability of a premutation allele in homozygous patients with myotonic dystrophy type I. Ann Neurol. 2002;52:435–41.
21. Kroksmark AK, Ekstrom AB, Bjorck E, Tulinius M. Myotonic dystrophy: muscle involvement in relation to disease type and size of expanded CTG-repeat sequence. Dev Med Child Neurol. 2005;47:478–85.

22. Tsilfidis C, MacKenzie AE, Mettler G, Barcelo J, Korneluk RG. Correlation between CTG trinucleotide repeat length and frequency of severe congenital myotonic dystrophy. Nat Genet. 1992;1:192–5.
23. Harley HG, Rundle SA, MacMillan JC, et al. Size of the unstable CTG repeat sequence in relation to phenotype and parental transmission in myotonic dystrophy. Am J Hum Genet. 1993;52:1164–74.
24. Lavedan C, Hofmann-Radvanyi H, Shelbourne P, et al. Myotonic dystrophy: size and sex-dependent dynamics of CTG meiotic instability and somatic mosaicism. Am J Hum Genet. 1993;52:873–83.
25. Redman JB, Fenwick Jr RG, Fu YH, Pizzuti A, Caskey CT. Relationship between parental trinucleotide CTG repeat length and severity of myotonic dystrophy in the offspring. JAMA. 1993;269:1960–5.
26. Hageman AT, Gabreels FJ, Liem KD, Renkawek K, Boon JM. Congenital myotonic dystrophy: a report on thirteen cases and a review of the literature. J Neurol Sci. 1993;115:95–101.
27. Casey EB, Aminoff MJ. Dystrophia myotonica presenting with dysphagia. Br Med J. 1971;2:443.
28. Dunn LJ, Dierker LI. Recurrent hydramnios in association with myotonia dystrophica. Obstet Gynecol. 1973;42:104–6.
29. Canavese F, Sussman MD. Orthopaedic manifestations of congenital myotonic dystrophy during childhood and adolescence. J Pediatr Orthop. 2009;29:208–13.
30. Mashiach R, Rimon E, Achiron R. Tent-shaped mouth as a presenting symptom of congenital myotonic dystrophy. Ultrasound Obstet Gynecol. 2002;20:312–3.
31. Sarnat HB, O'Connor T, Byrne PA. Clinical effects of myotonic dystrophy on pregnancy and the neonate. Arch Neurol. 1976;33:459–65.
32. Sjogreen L, Engvall M, Ekstrom AB, Lohmander A, Kiliaridis S, Tulinius M. Orofacial dysfunction in children and adolescents with myotonic dystrophy. Dev Med Child Neurol. 2007;49:18–22.
33. Campbell C, Sherlock R, Jacob P, Blayney M. Congenital myotonic dystrophy: assisted ventilation duration and outcome. Pediatrics. 2004;113:811–6.
34. Echenne B, Rideau A, Roubertie A, Sebire G, Rivier F, Lemieux B. Myotonic dystrophy type I in childhood Long-term evolution in patients surviving the neonatal period. Eur J Paediatr Neurol. 2008;12:210–23.
35. Modoni A, Silvestri G, Pomponi MG, Mangiola F, Tonali PA, Marra C. Characterization of the pattern of cognitive impairment in myotonic dystrophy type 1. Arch Neurol. 2004;61:1943–7.
36. Angeard N, Gargiulo M, Jacquette A, Radvanyi H, Eymard B, Heron D. Cognitive profile in childhood myotonic dystrophy type 1: is there global impairment? Neuromuscul Disord. 2007;17:451–8.
37. Di Costanzo A, Di Salle F, Santoro L, Bonavita V, Tedeschi G. Brain MRI features of congenital- and adult-form myotonic dystrophy type 1: case control study. Neuromuscul Disord. 2002;12:476–83.
38. Di Costanzo A, Santoro L, de Cristofaro M, Manganelli F, Di Salle F, Tedeschi G. Familial aggregation of white matter lesions in myotonic dystrophy type 1. Neuromuscul Disord. 2008;18:299–305.
39. Ekstrom AB, Hakenas-Plate L, Samuelsson L, Tulinius M, Wentz E. Autism spectrum conditions in myotonic dystrophy type 1: a study on 57 individuals with congenital and childhood forms. Am J Med Genet B Neuropsychiatr Genet. 2008;147B:918–26.
40. Douniol M, Jacquette A, Guilé JM, et al. Psychiatric and cognitive phenotype in children and adolescents with myotonic dystrophy. Eur Child Adolesc Psychiatry. 2009;18:705–15.
41. Steyaert J, de Die-Smulders C, Fryns JP, et al. Behavioral phenotype in childhood type of dystrophia myotonica. Am J Med Genet. 2000;96:888–9.
42. Bassez G, Lazarus A, Desguerre I, et al. Severe cardiac arrhythmias in young patients with myotonic dystrophy type 1. Neurology. 2004;63:1939–41.

43. Chebel S, Ben Hamda K, Boughammoura A, et al. Cardiac involvement in Steinert's myotonic dystrophy. Rev Neurol. 2005;161:932–9.
44. Delaporte C. Personality patterns in patients with myotonic dystrophy. Arch Neurol. 1998;55:635–40.
45. Winblad S, Lindberg C, Hansen S. Temperament and character in patients with classical myotonic dystrophy type 1 (DM-1). Neuromuscul Disord. 2005;15:287–92.
46. Thornton CA, Griggs RC, Moxley III RT. Myotonic dystrophy with no trinucleotide repeat expansion. Ann Neurol. 1994;35:269–72.
47. Day JW, Ricker K, Jacobsen JF, et al. Myotonic dystrophy type 2: molecular, diagnostic and clinical spectrum. Neurology. 2003;60:657–64.
48. Echenne B, Bassez G. Congenital and infantile myotonic dystrophy. Handb Clin Neurol. 2013;113:1387–93.
49. Day JW, Roelofs R, Leroy B, et al. Clinical and genetic characteristics of a five-generation family with a novel form of myotonic dystrophy (DM2). Neuromuscul Disord. 1999;9:19–27.
50. Ricker K, Koch MC, Lehmann-Horn F, et al. Proximal myotonic myopathy. Clinical features of a multisystem disorder similar to myotonic dystrophy. Arch Neurol. 1995;52:25–31.
51. Moxley III RT, Meola G, Udd B, et al. Report of the 84th ENMC workshop: PROMM (proximal myotonic myopathy) and other myotonic dystrophy-like syndromes: 2nd workshop. 13–15th October, 2000. Loosdrecht, The Netherlands. Neuromuscul Disord. 2002;12:306–17.
52. Schoser BG, Ricker K, Schneider-Gold C, et al. Sudden cardiac death in myotonic dystrophy type 2. Neurology. 2004;63:2402–4.
53. Meola G, Sansone V, Perani D, et al. Executive dysfunction and avoidant personality trait in myotonic dystrophy type 1 (DM1) and in proximal myotonic myopathy (DM2/PROMM). Neuromuscul Disord. 2003;13:813–21.
54. Savkur RS, Philips AV, Cooper TA, et al. Insulin receptor splicing alteration in myotonic dystrophy type 2. Am J Hum Genet. 2004;74:1309–13.
55. Anderson VB, McKenzie JA, Seton C, Fitzgerald DA, Webster RI, North KN, et al. Sniff nasal inspiratory pressure and sleep disordered breathing in childhood neuromuscular disorders. Neuromuscul Disord. 2012;22:528–33.
56. Vinereanu D, Bajaj BP, Fenton-May J, Rogers MT, Madler CF, Fraser AG. Subclinical cardiac involvement in myotonic dystrophy manifesting as decreased myocardial Doppler velocities. Neuromuscul Disord. 2004;14:188–94.
57. Botta A, Bonifazi E, Vallo L, et al. Italian guidelines for molecular analysis of myotonic dystrophies. Acta Myol. 2006;25:23–33.
58. Martorell L, Cobo AM, Baiget M, Naudo M, Poza JJ, Parra J. Prenatal diagnosis in myotonic dystrophy type 1. Thirteen years of experience: implications for reproductive counseling in DM1 families. Prenat Diagn. 2007;27:68–72.
59. Addis M, Serrenti M, Meloni C, Cau M, Melis MA. Triplet-primed PCR is more sensitive than southern blotting-long PCR for the diagnosis of myotonic dystrophy type1. Genet Test Mol Biomarkers. 2012;16:1428–31.
60. Kwiecinski H, Ryniewicz B, Ostrzycki A. Treatment of myotonia with antiarrhythmic drugs. Acta Neurol Scand. 1992;86:371–5.
61. Mostacciuolo ML, Miorin M, Martinello F, Angelini C, Perini P, Trevisan CP. Genetic epidemiology of congenital muscular dystrophy in a sample from north-east Italy. Hum Genet. 1996;97:277–9.
62. Hughes MI, Hicks EM, Nevin NC, Patterson VH. The prevalence of inherited neuromuscular disease in Northern Ireland. Neuromuscul Disord. 1996;6:69–73.
63. Darin N, Tulinius M. Neuromuscular disorders in childhood: a descriptive epidemiological study from western Sweden. Neuromuscul Disord. 2000;10:1–9.
64. Norwood FL, Harling C, Chinnery PF, Eagle M, Bushby K, Straub V. Prevalence of genetic muscle disease in northern England: in-depth analysis of a muscle clinic population. Brain. 2009;132:3175–86.

65. Bönnemann CG, Wang CH, Quijano-Roy S, Deconinck N, Bertini E, Ferreiro A, et al. Diagnostic approach to the congenital muscular dystrophies. Neuromuscul Disord. 2014;24:289–311.
66. Helbling-Leclerc A, Zhang X, Topaloglu H, et al. Mutations in the laminin alpha 2-chain gene (LAMA2) cause merosin-deficient congenital muscular dystrophy. Nat Genet. 1995;11:216–8.
67. Guicheney P, Vignier N, Helbling-Leclerc A, et al. Genetics of laminin alpha 2 chain (or merosin) deficient congenital muscular dystrophy: from identification of mutations to prenatal diagnosis. Neuromuscul Disord. 1997;7:180–6.
68. Philpot J, Cowan F, Pennock J, et al. Merosin-deficient congenital muscular dystrophy: the spectrum of brain involvement on magnetic resonance imaging. Neuromuscul Disord. 1999;9:81–5.
69. Muntoni F, Torelli S, Wells DJ, Brown SC. Muscular dystrophies due to glycosylation defects: diagnosis and therapeutic strategies. Curr Opin Neurol. 2011;24:437–42.
70. Wells L. The O-mannosylation pathway: glycosyltransferases and proteins implicated in congenital muscular dystrophy. J Biol Chem. 2013;288:6930–5.
71. Hara Y, Balci-Hayta B, Yoshida-Moriguchi T, et al. A dystroglycan mutation associated with limb-girdle muscular dystrophy. N Engl J Med. 2011;364:939–46.
72. Imbach T, Schenk B, Schollen E, et al. Deficiency of dolichol-phosphate-mannose synthase-1 causes congenital disorder of glycosylation type Ie. J Clin Invest. 2000;105:233–9.
73. Messina S, Tortorella G, Concolino D, et al. Congenital muscular dystrophy with defective alpha-dystroglycan, cerebellar hypoplasia, and epilepsy. Neurology. 2009;73:1599–601.
74. Yang AC, Ng BG, Moore SA, et al. Congenital disorder of glycosylation due to DPM1 mutations presenting with dystroglycanopathy-type congenital muscular dystrophy. Mol Genet Metab. 2013;110:345–51.
75. Brinas L, Richard P, Quijano-Roy S, et al. Early onset collagen VI myopathies: genetic and clinical correlations. Ann Neurol. 2010;68:511–20.
76. Bonnemann CG. The collagen VI-related myopathies: muscle meets its matrix. Nat Rev Neurol. 2011;7:379–90.
77. Nadeau A, Kinali M, Main M, et al. Natural history of Ullrich congenital muscular dystrophy. Neurology. 2009;73:25–31.
78. Foley AR, Quijano-Roy S, Collins J, et al. Natural history of pulmonary function in collagen VI-related myopathies. Brain. 2013;136:3625–33.
79. Yonekawa T, Komaki H, Okada M, et al. Rapidly progressive scoliosis and respiratory deterioration in Ullrich congenital muscular dystrophy. J Neurol Neurosurg Psychiatry. 2013;84:982–8.
80. Kirschner J, Hausser I, Zou Y, et al. Ullrich congenital muscular dystrophy: connective tissue abnormalities in the skin support overlap with Ehlers–Danlos syndromes. Am J Med Genet A. 2005;132:296–301.
81. Jurynec MJ, Xia R, Mackrill JJ, et al. Selenoprotein N is required for ryanodine receptor calcium release channel activity in human and zebrafish muscle. Proc Natl Acad Sci U S A. 2008;105:12485–90.
82. Arbogast S, Beuvin M, Fraysse B, Zhou H, Muntoni F, Ferreiro A. Oxidative stress in SEPN1-related myopathy: from pathophysiology to treatment. Ann Neurol. 2009;65:677–86.
83. Ferreiro A, Quijano-Roy S, Pichereau C, et al. Mutations of the selenoprotein N gene, which is implicated in rigid spine muscular dystrophy, cause the classical phenotype of multiminicore disease: reassessing the nosology of early-onset myopathies. Am J Hum Genet. 2002;71:739–49.
84. Schara U, Kress W, Bonnemann CG, et al. The phenotype and long-term follow-up in 11 patients with juvenile selenoprotein N1-related myopathy. Eur J Paediatr Neurol. 2008;12:224–30.
85. Scoto M, Cirak S, Mein R, et al. SEPN1-related myopathies: clinical course in a large cohort of patients. Neurology. 2011;76:2073–8.

86. Klein A, Lillis S, Munteanu I, Scoto M, Zhou H, Quinlivan R, et al. Clinical and genetic findings in a large cohort of patients with ryanodine receptor 1 gene-associated myopathies. Hum Mutat. 2012;33:981–8.

87. Bharucha-Goebel DX, Santi M, Medne L, Zukosky K, Zukosky K, Dastgir J, et al. Severe congenital ryr1-associated myopathy: The expanding clinicopathologic and genetic spectrum. Neurology. 2013;80:1584–9.

88. Rankin J, Ellard S. The laminopathies: a clinical review. Clin Genet. 2006;70:261–74.

89. Worman HJ, Ostlund C, Wang Y. Diseases of the nuclear envelope. Cold Spring Harb Perspect Biol. 2010;2:a000760.

90. D'Amico A, Haliloglu G, Richard P, et al. Two patients with 'Dropped head syndrome' due to mutations in LMNA or SEPN1 genes. Neuromuscul Disord. 2005;15:521–4.

91. Prigogine C, Richard P, Van den Bergh P, Groswasser J, Deconinck N. Novel LMNA mutation presenting as severe congenital muscular dystrophy. Pediatr Neurol. 2010;43:283–6.

92. Quijano-Roy S, Mbieleu B, Bonnemann CG, et al. De novo LMNA mutations cause a new form of congenital muscular dystrophy. Ann Neurol. 2008;64:177–86.

93. Nishino I, Kobayashi O, Goto Y, et al. A new congenital muscular dystrophy with mitochondrial structural abnormalities. Muscle Nerve. 1998;21:40–7.

94. Pegoraro E, Marks H, Garcia CA, Crawford T, Mancias P, Connolly AM, et al. Laminin alpha2 muscular dystrophy: genotype/phenotype studies of 22 patients. Neurology. 1998;51:101–10.

95. Nigro V, Savarese M. Genetic basis of limb-girdle muscular dystrophies: the 2014 update. Acta Myol. 2014;33:1–12.

96. Bashir R, Strachan T, Keers S, Stephenson A, Mahjneh I, Marconi G, et al. A gene for autosomal recessive limb-girdle muscular dystrophy maps to chromosome 2p. Hum Mol Genet. 1994;3:455–7.

97. Bejaoui K, Hirabayashi K, Hentati F, Haines JL, Ben Hamida C, Belal S, et al. Linkage of Miyoshi myopathy (distal autosomal recessive muscular dystrophy) locus to chromosome 2p12-14. Neurology. 1995;45:768–72.

98. Illa I, Serrano-Munuera C, Gallardo E, Lasa A, Rojas-García R, Palmer J, et al. Distal anterior compartment myopathy: a dysferlin mutation causing a new muscular dystrophy phenotype. Ann Neurol. 2001;49:130–4.

# Chapter 6
# Transition from Childhood to Adult in Patients with Muscular Dystrophy

**Elba Yesi Gerena Maldonado and Kathryn R. Wagner**

## Introduction

"We were the generation that was hoped for—and now we're here," announced L. Vance Taylor, a successful 36-year-old man with muscular dystrophy (Muscular Dystrophy Association (MDA) National Neuromuscular Transitions Summit, Washington D.C., September 23, 2011). In this one phrase, Mr. Taylor voices the current achievement and challenge that our healthcare system faces: an increasing adult population of patients with muscular dystrophy (MD) and a society that lacks the structure to support them.

In the past 30 years, we have seen an increase in the lifespan of patients with MDs especially those who have early onset of their disease [1]. The scientific and medical community has made great strides in the early care of patients with MDs and has published practice guidelines to promote better care for these patients [2, 3]. However, it has not been until recently that the community has started to address the quandary that is the transition phase from childhood to independent adulthood with complex medical conditions [4–7]. A survey done in the UK, where patients older than 15 years and their family members were interviewed from 2007 to 2009, showed that while advances in healthcare have increased life expectancy in patients with MDs, this has not been matched by an increase in support at home and in the community [4]. There is no doubt that the structured care coordination for pediatric patients with MDs is significantly different from the perceived lack of support these same individuals face once they become adults. The reason for this disparity is

E.Y. Gerena Maldonado, M.D. (✉)
Department of Rehabilitation Medicine, University of Washington,
1959 NE Pacific Street, Box 356490, Seattle, WA 98195-6490, USA
e-mail: egerena1@uw.edu

K.R. Wagner, M.D., Ph.D.
Kennedy Krieger Institute, Genetic and Muscle Diseases,
801 North Broadway, Baltimore, MD 21205, USA

© Springer International Publishing Switzerland 2015
R.A. Huml (ed.), *Muscular Dystrophy*, DOI 10.1007/978-3-319-17362-7_6

likely to be multifactorial; nevertheless, we need to start understanding the unique features of the transition period to develop effective strategies to maximize the likelihood of success in adult life.

This challenge is not unique to the field of MD. The National Alliance to Advance Adolescent Health estimates that chronic health conditions affect approximately 25% of the 18 million U.S. young adults ages 18–21, who should be transitioning to adult-centered healthcare. Each year, approximately 750,000 young people in the U.S. with special healthcare need transition to adult care [8]. The fields of cystic fibrosis, perinatally acquired HIV, and pediatric organ transplantation are just three examples that have similarly needed to adjust their thinking and prepare their patients for an adult life where, previously, there was none.

Our goal with this chapter is to highlight the importance of the transition period in the life of an individual with MD and to provide helpful resources available for guidance and support.

## Emerging Adulthood

Emerging adulthood has been defined as "the period when often people explore a variety of possible life directions in love, work, and worldviews... where the scope of independent exploration of life's possibilities is greater for most people than it will be at any other period of the life course" [9]. It is usually during this period when people start to mold their personalities and define themselves in their community. Therefore, it is of the upmost importance that our society provides the adequate groundwork on which young adults, especially those with disabilities, can establish and design their own life stories.

There are various psychological models of development that have been put forward to explain the key stages in an adolescent's life. Some of these models describe this period as filled with change in which young adults are assuming new roles in all facets of their lives. They can experience conflicting feelings between the excitement about the prospect of autonomy and the sense of abandonment due to the previous dependent nature of their relationships with their parents and/or caregivers [10].

The literature suggests that relationships with parents remain the most influential of all adolescent relationships [11], and their support has been associated with good outcomes [12]. During this period, the parents need to talk frequently with their child about his/her interests so that a transition plan can be built upon these interests. The parents need to familiarize themselves with various local and state agencies and file for appropriate services. Most importantly, the parents need to foster and not limit their child's dreams.

Previous research has mainly focused on retrospective post-transition interviews, and less is known about younger adolescents and their families as they approach the transition period. Given the complexity of the arrangements in which these children grow up, addressing all of their needs at the same time is a challenging task. Moreover, it can be counterproductive in the end, as it can be overwhelming for these young adults to be made responsible for all of their healthcare needs in a short amount of time. Their care should be introduced as a step-by-step process where they are included in decision making, information sharing, while at the same time their parents remain informed and involved. In a study done in Denmark in 2011, 16 young adults with cystic fibrosis were interviewed about their transition experience. One of the highlighted points in this study was that these patients preferred to have a gradual transfer of responsibility of their own medical care during their young adulthood [13]. Similarly, experts in Duchenne muscular dystrophy (DMD) urge that transition not be thought of as a single event, but as a continuing process of increased choices and autonomy [5].

## Timetable for Growing Up

Parents and physicians may differ in their perceptions of when to begin teaching children about self-management of their healthcare. The mean age identified by parents is 12 years, while that of pediatricians is 9.5 years [11]. So, the question remains, when should we start the transition period for children with physical disabilities, in particular those with MDs?

Due to each child's unique circumstances, it would not be prudent to stipulate a definitive age when parents should start the conversation of transition with their child. Nevertheless, preparation must begin early enough to ensure adolescents develop the knowledge and skills to take ownership of their chronic illness and disease management in an effective manner.

Some of the most common methods that are being used to start the transition stage have been the implementation of "timetables for growing up". These transition plans have some variability in their designs; nonetheless, most agree that certain "transition topics" should start to be discussed around the ages of 12–13 years. For example, the timetable provided by the Holland Bloorview Kids Rehabilitation Hospital or the MDA's "Road Map to Independence," which encourages conversations about topics of human development and social interactions when the child is at the pre-to-early adolescent stage. Once they reach the mid-to-late teens, the timetables focus on developing independent living skills (e.g. contributing to discussions and decisions regarding their medical treatments, being assigned chores around the house, driving vs. public transportation as means of mobility, etc.). Topics like future career goals should also be addressed in a timely manner, as it has been found in the literature that children with disabilities worldwide tend to be excluded from certain schooling subjects (due to lower rates of school attendance given their multiple medical appointments and lower transition rates to higher levels of education) when compared to kids without physical and/or cognitive impairments [14]. Exclusion from education has an immediate impact on a child in terms of exclusion from social participation, reduced personal well-being and welfare, and likely dependence on caregivers.

## Commencement of Transition Years

The parents' approaches to promoting health and well-being for their adolescents with physical disabilities tend to be diverse. Some see themselves as the primary source of information; others rely solely on school, while a few others view friends and the media as a resource. Some parents have expressed concerns and anxiety about the fact that they believe that their adolescent with a physical disability is going to encounter greater difficulties in relationships and sexual expression [15]. All of these factors will influence the outcomes of the transition period in patients with physical and/or cognitive disabilities. Given the dual role of the parents as both progenitors and caregivers for these children, the literature has described the tendency of these parents to be overprotective [16]. However, another explanation for their "overprotection" during the transition period is that their behavior is a deliberate strategy to provide their adolescent with more time and energy for school and friends.

Nevertheless, the goal of the transition years is to promote the development of skills for independence in multiple facets of the teenager's life. One of the major concerns that parents of children with disabilities have is the development of a healthy social life and integration into their community [4]. Parents have dual worries of how their children will cope with the changes that all human beings go through while growing up and at the same time adding to the process the complexity of their physical disabilities. It is for this reason that both health providers and caregivers should address socialization of adolescents and young adults prior to them reaching adulthood.

It is important for patients with MDs to feel that they are an integral part of society. At the same time, they benefit from certain events or activities where their physical disabilities are normalized. Several organizations provide free camp experiences for those with MD. The MDA organizes a one-week summer camp for children and young adults (ages 6–17) where they can meet other youth with a variety of neuromuscular disorders and share their life experiences (http://mda.org/summer-camp). The Jett Foundation offers a week-long "Camp Promise" for those with MD (https://www.camppromise.org/). If the young adult is interested in the fine arts (music, theatre, visual arts), there are programs like the International Organization on Arts and Disability providing career building opportunities in the arts both nationally and internationally (http://www.kennedy-center.org/education/vsa/).

## *Self-Advocacy*

Being a strong self-advocate is necessary for the youth with MD. No one will understand his/her particular manifestations of disease and resulting needs as well. Being able to effectively communicate these needs, propose solutions for how they should be met, and engage others in these solutions are key factors in success.

As emerging adults, a balance should be struck between establishing independence and receiving support from parents/ caregivers. These young adults need to have a good understanding of their condition, be it a fast or slowly progressive MD. Health literacy is a priority.

There are multiple opportunities for the youth to become an advocate for the MD community. Local groups sponsored by the MDA provided supportive environments for discussion and activities. If the adolescent is interested in groups that are focused on their own specific diagnosis, there are various groups which provide information and support: PPMD for Duchenne and Becker muscular dystrophy, FSHD Society and the Friends of FSH for FSHD, and the Myotonic Dystrophy Foundation, for myotonic dystrophy, to name a few (websites provided below).

## *Social*

In this era of globalization that has risen from the advances in the telecommunications infrastructure, it is easy to acquire large amounts of information, some of which might not be necessarily correct or appropriate for certain age groups. It is for this reason that certain topics should not be taboo at home or school and should be addressed by a trustworthy adult. Children are exposed to subjects like smoking, drug use, and alcohol on a daily basis. Topics related to sexuality, contraception, and preconception counseling and surveillance should also be addressed. The existing literature is scarce in research concerning sexual health and MDs [17]. Openness and knowledge are integral for a successful rapport with the adolescent with MDs seeking counsel in these matters. Common barriers that affect the success of these talks are the sensitivity of the subject matter, the parents' insecurity in how they can be supportive, or the parents' abdication of the discussion of sexual health to someone else.

The adolescents themselves might be reluctant to initiate communication about sexual health problems, especially if they believe that the adult is unavailable to offer support or if they believe that they shouldn't be sexually active due to their disability. It is for this reason that they should have a support group identified which can reliably provide additional accurate information and advice.

Young adults are faced with a world that increasingly is more available through different communication devices. Although these devices, such as computers and mobile devices, can be used as assistive devices for communication, they might also promote isolation. The social integration in the community cannot be overemphasized, given the fact that the natural history of growing up is that certain childhood friendships grow apart as kids become teenagers and eventually adults.

## *Education*

The Individuals with Disabilities Education Act (IDEA) provides federal financial assistance to state and local educational agencies to ensure that students with disabilities receive an education "designed to meet their unique needs and prepare them for employment and independent living" (http://idea.ed.gov/explore/home). IDEA was reauthorized in 2004 with very specific language about transition planning. One of the primary methods by which IDEA is enacted is through Individual Education Programs (IEPS). It is imperative that children with MDs be gradually integrated in the parent–teacher meetings about their education. They should be aware of what their IEP entails, and how it is being tailored to not only their physical needs but also their academic interests. They should talk openly about the careers that they want to pursue and explore opportunities with volunteer work or part-time jobs.

By the time students are starting high-school, they should be contacting the Disability Support Services Office of various post-secondary schools. Students need to self-identify and self-advocate whether they choose a vocational school, community college, or university. There is a wide range of accommodations made for post-secondary students with disabilities from schools such as Edinboro University in Pennsylvania (www.edinboro.edu), which has dozens of students making use of attendant care, meal aides, homework aides, and on-campus wheelchair repair services to the majority of colleges which are barely wheelchair accessible [18]. Several universities and colleges provide opportunities for students with disabilities to have exposure to future employers. Programs like the DO-IT (http://www.washington.edu/doit), based at the University Of Washington College Of Engineering, help in bringing together students and employers in a setting that can provide career advancement for these patients. The process for university students to acquire or receive services tends to be determined by how proactive students are to advocate for themselves and provide clear documentation of the disability. A self-advocating student in a college with a strong Disability Support Services Office is a combination that yields a safe and rewarding new home transitioning from the parents' home to complete independence.

## *Self-Care*

Mastering normal developmental tasks, such as household chores or an after-school job, can help boost the self-confidence and independence of an adolescent with MD. As the child begins to manifest more autonomy, a clinical checklist updated on each visit prompts review and discussion of the patient's progress toward self-management and eventual transition.

By the time the child is in the pre-teen to early teenage years, conversations about future living situations should be brought to the table. They should be slowly progressed to learn independent living skills. They should also practice budgeting and banking skills. Some clinics provide counseling with social workers or case managers that are able to guide the family in regard to community resources for their children.

Many states offer transition programs and services to help prepare individuals with a developmental disability to gain employment and independent living. These services may include employment counseling, employment training, assistive technology, and independent living skills training. There is wide variability in the number, types, and funding of these services across the nation.

## Transition to Adult Healthcare

A well-organized and well-timed transition from child-oriented to adult-oriented healthcare allows young people to optimize their ability to assume adult roles and functioning in society. For many young people with special healthcare needs, this will mean a transfer from a pediatric to an adult healthcare professional; for many others, it will involve an ongoing relationship with the same provider but with a reorientation of clinical interactions. With a successful transition, healthcare is uninterrupted, function is maximized, and morbidity and mortality are reduced. There are several challenges, however, to obtaining uninterrupted healthcare services during the transition period. These include the lack of a formalized transfer linkage between pediatric and adult medical services, which frequently leaves patients and families to personally assemble their own adult medicine team. A consensus statement of the American Academy of Pediatrics, the American Academy of Family Practice, and the American College of Physicians recommended a written heathcare transition plan by age 14 but in the experience of the authors, such a plan is rare from MD providers [7]. Unfortunately, pediatric patients lose their medical safety net at the same time that they are losing a social safety net, that of their secondary school and the services that it often provides.

Pediatric and adult healthcare systems are structured differently. Children are frequently cared for at children's hospitals equipped with multiple disciplines, which not only include their physicians, but also include social services, education, vocational training, and recreation. The processes of teaching them to take responsibility for their own healthcare needs are vital, as they will need to become their own advocates once they transition to adult healthcare. Some of the adult neuromuscular medicine clinics also provide services that include assessment, consultation, and intervention from various disciplines including physiatrists/neurologists, cardiologists, pulmonologists, occupational therapists, physiotherapists, social workers, and genetic counselors. However, in a survey of patients with adult MD, they were more likely to receive services from fewer health professionals and were less satisfied with their current healthcare compared to when they were children, which was often associated with a decline in health outcomes [4].

Successful transition from pediatric to adult medicine can be achieved by multiple different strategies. Some healthcare institutions have both adult and pediatric clinics where the transition is seamless with the youth being able to meet his new team prior to full transition, records staying in the same facility, and some specialists remaining the same person. Programs such as those in children's hospitals, which include a complete transfer of care at age 18 or 21, are implementing transition care programs that involve some continuity with the pediatric physician following transition to the adult team. There are a few examples of formal transition planning that adhered to national policy guidelines [7].

Improving clinical care for young adults with MD is one of the current objectives for the adult healthcare system. Advisory committees composed of those MD patients who have already navigated the transition process and suffered the consequences of a healthcare system not equipped for them are being developed to help identify barriers to accessing appropriate healthcare services needed for future generations. Among the areas that have been identified that need to be addressed, one of the most urgent ones is the facilitation of follow-up and referrals and enhancement of community linkages for services.

## Conclusion

We have all witnessed that the lack of a carefully orchestrated transition plan results in a deterioration in the quality of life of young adults with MDs. However, those few who have been able to have a successful transition have attained skills necessary to manage their own personal needs and healthcare. They are effective self-advocates and are able to pursue their own interests. They have assembled knowledgeable and responsive medical teams who work diligently to free them from recurrent illnesses, pain, and hospitalizations. They find the balance between independence and the need for social/physical support in their lives acceptable. Our goal is to make these examples the norm of all young adults with MD who are transitioning into adulthood.

It is imperative that the MD community continues to work on strengthening the transition process to ensure success of the upcoming generations. Some clear current barriers are inadequate communication between pediatric and adult providers, an adult healthcare system unprepared to meet the various needs of these often complicated patients, the lack of integration of social services at the local and state level, and the scarcity of job opportunities for those with disabilities. There are fortunately several groups, such as those listed below, as well as governmental agencies that are highly invested in improving transition for youths. In addition, with proper guidance, these young men and women are likely to positively shape the environment for themselves and for the next generation.

Useful websites for young adults with MDs:

- http://hollandbloorview.ca/programsandservices/ProgramsServicesAZ/Growingupready/TimetableforGrowingUp
- http://transitions.mda.org/
- http://mda.org/summer-camp

- http://www.kennedy-center.org/education/vsa/
- http://www.bristol.ac.uk/norahfry/research/completed-projects/ecominganadult.pdf
- http://www.doe.virginia.gov/special_ed/transition_svcs/outcomes_project/college_guide.pdf
- https://www.dshs.wa.gov/jjra/division-vocational-rehabilitation
- https://www.dshs.wa.gov/dda
- http://wid.org/publications/downloads/Latinos%20with%20Dis.%20-%20Spanish.pdf

# References

1. Eagle M, et al. Survival in Duchenne muscular dystrophy: improvements in life expectancy since 1967 and the impact of home nocturnal ventilation. Neuromuscul Disord. 2002;12(10): 926–9.
2. Bushby K, et al. Diagnosis and management of Duchenne muscular dystrophy, part 2: implementation of multidisciplinary care. Lancet Neurol. 2010;9(2):177–89.
3. Turner C, Hilton-Jones D. Myotonic dystrophy: diagnosis, management and new therapies. Curr Opin Neurol. 2014;27(5):599–606.
4. Abbott D, Carpenter J, Bushby K. Transition to adulthood for young men with Duchenne muscular dystrophy: research from the UK. Neuromuscul Disord. 2012;22(5):445–6.
5. Schrans DG, et al. Transition in Duchenne muscular dystrophy: an expert meeting report and description of transition needs in an emergent patient population (Parent Project Muscular Dystrophy Transition Expert Meeting 17–18 June 2011, Amsterdam, The Netherlands). Neuromuscul Disord. 2013;23(3):283–6.
6. Rahbek J, et al. Adult life with Duchenne muscular dystrophy: observations among an emerging and unforeseen patient population. Pediatr Rehabil. 2005;8(1):17–28.
7. American Academy of Pediatrics, American Academy of Family Physicians, American College of Physicians-American Society of Internal Medicine. A consensus statement on health care transitions for young adults with special health care needs. Pediatrics. 2002;110(6 Pt 2):1304–6.
8. Goodman DM, et al. Adults with chronic health conditions originating in childhood: inpatient experience in children's hospitals. Pediatrics. 2011;128(1):5–13.
9. Arnett JJ. Emerging adulthood. A theory of development from the late teens through the twenties. Am Psychol. 2000;55(5):469–80.
10. Nakhla M, et al. Transition to adult care for youths with diabetes mellitus: findings from a Universal Health Care System. Pediatrics. 2009;124(6):e1134–41.
11. Slap GB. Adolescent medicine. The requisites in pediatrics, xix. Philadelphia: Mosby/Elsevier; 2008. p. 330.
12. Kyngas H, Rissanen M. Support as a crucial predictor of good compliance of adolescents with a chronic disease. J Clin Nurs. 2001;10(6):767–74.
13. Bregnballe V, Schiotz PO, Lomborg K. Parenting adolescents with cystic fibrosis: the adolescents' and young adults' perspectives. Patient Prefer Adherence. 2011;5:563–70.
14. Kuper H, et al. The impact of disability on the lives of children; cross-sectional data including 8,900 children with disabilities and 898,834 children without disabilities across 30 countries. PLoS One. 2014;9(9):e107300.
15. Antle BJ, et al. An exploratory study of parents' approaches to health promotion in families of adolescents with physical disabilities. Child Care Health Dev. 2008;34(2):185–93.

16. Holmbeck GN, et al. Observed and perceived parental overprotection in relation to psychosocial adjustment in preadolescents with a physical disability: the mediational role of behavioral autonomy. J Consult Clin Psychol. 2002;70(1):96–110.
17. Areskoug-Josefsson K. Muscular dystrophy and sexual health. OA Musculoskelet Med. 2013;1(2):17.
18. Tiedemann CW. College success for students with physical disabilities. Austin: Prufrock Press; 2012.

# Chapter 7
# Overview of Current Treatments for Muscular Dystrophy

**Zheng (Jane) Fan**

## Introduction

As described in earlier chapters, muscular dystrophy (MD) refers to a group of hereditary diseases characterized by progressive wasting of skeletal muscles, often related to muscle membranes or supporting proteins. Current treatment is focused on symptomatic management and rehabilitation, and monitoring for disease complications. There is no cure for MD; however, better patient care especially with multidisciplinary approach has reduced mortality and morbidity significantly.

This chapter discusses general management strategies for MD and also describes treatments for the following subtypes of MDs: dystrophinopathies [Duchenne muscular dystrophy (DMD) and Becker muscular dystrophy (BMD)], Facioscapulohumeral muscular dystrophy (FSHD), myotonic dystrophy, and limb girdle muscular dystrophy (LGMD).

## Diagnosis and Initial Evaluation

Accurate diagnosis is important as a first step for managing MD. This is contingent on a targeted history and examination, biochemical, and genetic testing; sometimes with additional testing such as muscle biopsy, neurophysiological assessment, and muscle imaging. Muscle biopsy used to be the gold standard; however, it is increasingly replaced by genetic testing. The detection rate with genetic testing for DMD and BMD is ~95% using deletion/duplication study and reflex to sequencing

Z. (Jane) Fan, M.D. (✉)
Department of Neurology, University of North Carolina at Chapel Hill,
CB# 7025, 2145 Physicians Office Bldg., 170 Manning Drive, Chapel Hill,
NC 27599-7025, USA
e-mail: zhengfan@med.unc.edu

© Springer International Publishing Switzerland 2015
R.A. Huml (ed.), *Muscular Dystrophy*, DOI 10.1007/978-3-319-17362-7_7

analysis if deletion/duplication study is negative [1]. The genetic basis for FSHD has been elucidated in recent decades, and the genetic testing detection rate is ~95% for patients with FSHD where a contraction mutation of the D4Z4 macrosatellite array in the subtelomeric region of chromosome 4q35 can be identified [2]. Next generation sequencing technology such as whole exome sequencing (WES) has significantly improved our ability to diagnose subtypes of LGMD, as the traditional sequencing method limits testing to one gene at a time. While electromyography and nerve conduction studies have been a traditional part of the assessment of a patient with MD, these tests are not believed to be indicated or necessary for diagnosis unless other means are inconclusive. Muscle imaging is becoming more widely accepted as it is noninvasive and various forms of MD often result in unique patterns. This approach is also very sensitive, enabling inflammatory myopathies (also called myositis) and metabolic myopathies — which may mimic MD but require different management — to be ruled out. For these conditions, specific treatments exist and accurate early diagnosis improves outcomes.

It is also worth mentioning that some subtypes of MD, such as myotonic dystrophy, are often missed in the presentation. Hilbert et al. found that patients with myotonic dystrophy type 1 (DM1) experienced an average of seven years delay to diagnosis, and members with myotonic dystrophy type 2 (DM2) had an even more stunning delay of 14 years before receiving a correct diagnosis [3]. Thus, the importance of clinical suspicion from clinicians and families cannot be overestimated.

# Management of MDs

## Overall Strategies

A multidisciplinary team approach has changed the landscape for the treatment of MD and represents the standard of care. Despite the lack of cures, improved supportive care has improved the life span of patients with MDs. One example is that patients with Duchenne MD lived on average until their late teens in the 1950s; today, they typically live until their late twenties and thirties, which is largely attributable to better supportive care. This may include noninvasive ventilation during the day, and at night, orthopedic care and preventive measures [4, 5]. Clinicians should refer patients with MD to a clinic that has access to multiple specialties designed to care for patients with neuromuscular disorders [6].

## Specific Therapy

Very few subtypes of MD have specific treatments. Examples are corticosteroids for DMD and treatment for myotonia in myotonic dystrophy type 1 (DM1).

Corticosteroids are the only medication currently available that slows the decline in muscle strength and function in DMD. These drugs are estimated to prolong ambulation by an average of approximately two years. However, corticosteroids are associated with many side effects, especially with long-term use. The optimal age for starting corticosteroids is under investigation in a randomized double-blind trial (Clinicaltrials.gov, NCT01603407, PIs Robert Griggs MD and Kate Bushby, MD). It should be noted that corticosteroids are not indicated for BMD or LGMD.

Myotonia in DM1 is typically mild to moderate and rarely requires treatment [7]. Anecdotally, some individuals have responded to mexilitene or carbamazepine. Logigian and colleagues found mexilitene 150–200 mg TID effective and safe for treating myotonia [8].

Supplements such as coenzyme Q10, carnitine, and antioxidants sometimes are used by families and clinicians. There is not enough evidence to make recommendations.

## Cardiac Management

Cardiac muscles resemble skeletal muscles in some ways, and many, though not all, forms of MD have associated cardiac involvement, which is a major cause for mortality and morbidity. The main cardiac involvements are progressive cardiomyopathy and/or cardiac arrhythmia. Patients with MD with cardiac involvements often do not have symptoms such as chest pain or pedal edema, but are often identified only by cardiac testing. Angiotensin-converting enzyme (ACE) inhibitors are the first line for managing cardiomyopathy. Pacemakers can be life-saving in MD with cardiac arrhythmia, especially in Emery–Dreifuss muscular dystrophy (EDMD) and myotonic dystrophy type I. Regular monitoring of cardiac function using echocardiogram, EKG, and cardiac Holter monitoring are indicated and early referral to cardiologist is highly recommended.

## Respiratory Management

The majority of forms of MD are associated with oropharyngeal and/or ventilator muscle weakness, which predispose patients to respiratory failure, which is a major cause of mortality and morbidity in MD. The diaphragm is a skeletal muscle, and weakness plays a significant role in respiratory failure in MD patients. Patients with respiratory failure often do not have symptoms such as dyspnea, which typically precede the onset of respiratory failure. Patients with respiratory failure secondary to muscle weakness in MD often have improved quality of life and outcomes with noninvasive pulmonary ventilation [9, 10]. Early monitoring using a lung function test and referral to pulmonologist is important.

## Sleep Disorder Management

Sleep disorders in MD patients are under-recognized, as these patients often do not present with excessive daytime sleepiness, and fatigue is often attributed to the MD itself. Diaphragm weakness makes patients with MD at greater risk during certain sleep stages such as rapid eye movement (REM) sleep, which relies on the diaphragm for ventilation. Sleep-related hypoventilation often precedes daytime hypoventilation.

Our preliminary data show that patients with DMD have sleep-related hypoventilation without clinical symptoms. Patients with MD are also at risk of obstructive sleep apnea (OSA) due to upper airway muscle weakness and obesity that is more prevalent in MD due to reduced activity level and corticosteroid usage. Both sleep-related hypoventilation and OSA can be effectively treated with PAP therapy and treatment improves outcome and quality of life. High clinical suspicion and overnight sleep study (polysomnography) should be considered in MD patients with considerable weakness, especially in those who are non-ambulatory.

## Rehabilitative Management

The goal for rehabilitative management is to maintain mobility and functional independence for as long as possible, with a focus on maximizing quality of life. Patients should have periodic assessments by physical and occupational therapists who are familiar with MD, including symptomatic and preventive screenings. Bracing and assistive devices are adapted to the patient's deficiencies and contracture, in order to preserve mobility and function and prevent contractures. With the advancement of electric wheelchairs and assistive devices, non-ambulatory patients with MD are often able to preserve a certain degree of independence and quality of life [11, 12].

In general, low-intensity aerobic exercise and strength training are recommended. Swimming is often recommended and especially enjoyed by non-ambulatory patients with MD. Swimming uses upper extremity muscles and truncal muscles that are not used much by routine aerobic exercise. There are concerns about exercise-induced muscle damage and myoglobinuria following supramaximal high-intensity exercise [13].

## Orthopedic Management

Spinal deformities, such as scoliosis, kyphosis, and rigid spine, can occur in subtypes of MD. These deformities can result in pain and functional impairment, such as interfering with pulmonary function. Patients with spinal deformity and foot contractures should be referred to orthopedic surgeons for monitoring and surgical interventions if deemed necessary [4].

Winging of the scapula can be common in subtypes of MD such as FSHD and EDMD. The benefit of scapular fixation surgery is debatable. There is no evidence from randomized trials to support the suggestion from observational studies that operative interventions produce significant benefits. However, this has to be balanced against postoperative immobilization, the need for physiotherapy, and potential complications [14].

## Nutrition

Patients with MD may have difficulty receiving adequate oral food intake due to dysphagia or inability to feed themselves linked to arm weakness. Maintaining adequate nutrition and body weight is important for optimizing strength, function, and quality of life. When oral food intake is inadequate, other means of maintaining intake (e.g., gastrostomy or jejunostomy feeding tubes) may be needed to maintain optimal nutrition [4, 6].

## Psychosocial Management

In addition to its medical burden, MD may be associated with marked psychosocial stress for patients and their families. Assessments are targeted at the areas of emotional adjustment and coping, neurocognitive functioning, possible autism spectrum disorder, depression, and social support [4]. Referral to a psychologist and psychiatrist should be made if concerns are identified. Children with DMD often highly appreciate activities such as "Make a Wish" trips. Families with MD also benefit from useful resources provided by foundations such as the Muscular Dystrophy Association (MDA), Parent Project Muscular Dystrophy (PPMD), TREAT NMD, and the FSH society.

Palliative care is important part of care for subtypes of MD patients in later stages of the disease. This not only provides pain control, but also includes emotional and spiritual support, assists families in clarifying treatment goals and making difficult treatment decisions, and addresses issues related to grief and bereavement [4].

## Genetic Counseling and Preventive Measures

Genetic counseling is the process of providing individuals and families with information on the nature, inheritance, and implications of genetic disorders, to help them make informed medical and personal decisions. All forms of MD are genetic disorders, either inherited from parents or as a de novo event. Risks to family members should be assessed. Options such as prenatal testing should be offered to female carriers. All patients with MD should be referred for genetic counseling after diagnosis.

The risk of malignant hyperthermia in patients with MD is a concern for families. Gurnaney and colleagues did not find an increased risk of malignant hyperthermia susceptibility in patients with DMD or BMD compared with the general population. However, dystrophic patients who are exposed to inhaled anesthetics may develop disease-related cardiac complications, or rarely, a malignant hyperthermia-like syndrome characterized by rhabdomyolysis. This latter complication may also occur postoperatively. Succinylcholine administration is associated with life-threatening hyperkalemia and should be avoided in patients with DMD and BMD [13]. It is important for patients with MD to discuss malignant hyperthermia-like risk with the anesthesiologist in any pre-op assessment.

## *Therapies Under Investigation*

MD is an area of active research, including multiple clinical trials. Updated information can be found by searching the www.clinicaltrials.gov website. Despite many trials in progress, such as exon skipping for DMD patients with certain genotypes (DMD exon 50 deletion), none has yet successfully completed registration trials. Several approaches for patients with LGMD, such as gene therapy, myoblast transplantation, neutralizing antibody to myostatin, and growth hormone, have promise, but clinical evaluation is not yet complete [6].

## Summary

MD comprises a group of heterogeneous genetic conditions with progressive skeletal muscle weakness. Despite the fact that there is no cure for MD, a multidisciplinary team approach with supportive care, such as noninvasive ventilation, improves outcomes including life span and quality of life.

## References

1. Darras B, Miller D, Urion D. Dystrophinopathies. In: Pagon R, Adam M, Ardinger H, editors. GeneReviews® [Internet], vol. 1993–2014. Seattle: University of Washington; 2014.
2. Lemmers R, Miller D, van der Maarel S. Facioscapulohumeral muscular dystrophy. In: Pagon R, Adam M, Ardinger H, editors. GeneReviews® [Internet]. Seattle: University of Washington; 2014.
3. Hilbert JE, Ashizawa T, Day JW, Luebbe EA, Martens WB, McDermott MP, et al. Diagnostic odyssey of patients with myotonic dystrophy. J Neurol. 2013;260:2497–504.

4. Bushby K, Finkel R, Birnkrant DJ, Case LE, Clemens PR, Cripe L, et al. Diagnosis and management of Duchenne muscular dystrophy, part 2: implementation of multidisciplinary care. Lancet Neurol. 2010;9:177–89.
5. Bushby K, Finkel R, Birnkrant DJ, Case LE, Clemens PR, Cripe L, et al. Diagnosis and management of Duchenne muscular dystrophy, part 1: diagnosis, and pharmacological and psychosocial management. Lancet Neurol. 2010;9:77–93.
6. Narayanaswami P, Weiss M, Selcen D, David W, Raynor E, Carter G, et al. Evidence-based guideline summary: diagnosis and treatment of limb-girdle and distal dystrophies: report of the guideline development subcommittee of the American Academy of Neurology and the practice issues review panel of the American Association of Neuromuscular & Electrodiagnostic Medicine. Neurology. 2014;83:1453–63.
7. Ricker K. Myotonic dystrophy and proximal myotonic myopathy. J Neurol. 1999;246:334–8.
8. Logigian EL, Martens WB, Moxley RT, McDermott MP, Dilek N, Wiegner AW, et al. Mexiletine is an effective antimyotonia treatment in myotonic dystrophy type 1. Neurology. 2010;74:1441–8.
9. Benditt JO, Boitano LJ. Pulmonary issues in patients with chronic neuromuscular disease. Am J Respir Crit Care Med. 2013;187:1046–55.
10. Villanova M, Brancalion B, Mehta AD. Duchenne muscular dystrophy: life prolongation by noninvasive ventilatory support. Am J Phys Med Rehabil. 2014;93:595–9.
11. Miller RG, Jackson CE, Kasarskis EJ, England JD, Forshew D, Johnston W, et al. Practice parameter update: the care of the patient with amyotrophic lateral sclerosis: multidisciplinary care, symptom management, and cognitive/behavioral impairment (an evidence-based review): report of the Quality Standards Subcommittee of the American Academy of Neurology. Neurology. 2009;73:1227–33.
12. Aitkens SG, McCrory MA, Kilmer DD, Bernauer EM. Moderate resistance exercise program: its effect in slowly progressive neuromuscular disease. Arch Phys Med Rehabil. 1993;74:711–5.
13. Gurnaney H, Brown A, Litman RS. Malignant hyperthermia and muscular dystrophies. Anesth Analg. 2009;109:1043–8.
14. Orrell, RW, Copeland, S, and Rose, MR. Scapular fixation in muscular dystrophy. Cochrane Database Syst Rev. 2010;CD003278. doi:10.1002/14651858.CD003278.pub2.

# Chapter 8
# Physical Therapy and Orthotic Devices

Laura E. Case

## Introduction

Muscular dystrophies (MDs) are a group of genetically based neuromuscular disorders characterized by disease-specific patterns of progressive muscle weakness accompanied by postural compensations and the risk of progressive contracture, deformity, and compromised function which may be accompanied by involvement across numerous body systems [1–14]. Individual MDs differ in the genetic basis, the cause and site of pathology, specific clinical features, distribution and extent of involvement, natural history, and prognosis [15–18], the details of which have been covered in previous chapters.

Similarities in the clinical presentation of MDs have allowed the use of common principles of clinical management and intervention in the provision of optimal comprehensive care with the coordinated expertise of a multidisciplinary team [5, 6, 19, 20]. Comprehensive, anticipatory physical therapy (PT) management of MD is based upon an understanding of the pathokinesiology of each type of MD, an understanding of the progression of the pathokinesiology over time, individual evaluation within the context of each individual's life and goals, and provision of consistent, preventative management across the lifespan in order to minimize the clinical and functional impact of the diagnosis and to optimize quality of life [1–3, 5, 6, 11, 19–24].

Historically, physical therapists have worked with individuals with MDs to minimize the clinical impact of the cellular pathology, to prevent secondary

L.E. Case, D.P.T., M.S., P.C.S., C./N.D.T. (✉)
Division of Physical Therapy, Department of Community and Family Medicine,
Duke University Medical Center, DUMC Box 104002, Durham, NC 27708, USA
e-mail: laura.case@duke.edu

© Springer International Publishing Switzerland 2015
R.A. Huml (ed.), *Muscular Dystrophy*, DOI 10.1007/978-3-319-17362-7_8

complications, to promote and maintain the maximum level of function and functional independence, and to achieve and maintain the highest possible quality of life for all individuals in spite of the disease process and/or progression [6, 25–28].

We are now entering an exciting new era, in which the natural histories of neuromuscular disorders are changing and improving based on improved medical care and management, and in which actual disease modifying treatments are emerging (see Chapter 4). PT management may increasingly, and for the first time, have the opportunity to assist in contributing to improvement and recovery in individuals with muscle diseases in addition to using prospective anticipatory care to manage impairments and optimize function and participation. In this new era, it will remain important to understand and continue to use optimal principles of intervention in comprehensive, anticipatory, preventative management and to optimize the benefits of disease modifying treatments as they emerge.

## Pathokinesiology

The underlying genetic basis and cellular pathology that characterize specific MDs differ, but each is typically characterized by a unique and genetically based progressive degeneration of muscle often accompanied by fibrosis and fatty infiltration that contributes to the development of contracture and deformity [29] (see Chapters 3–5). A self-perpetuating cycle of events in MDs has been described [14], in which imbalanced muscle weakness, compensatory movement patterns and postural habits, and the influence of gravity interact in the progression of disability [1, 2, 11, 14, 19, 30–32]. Weakness often progresses proximal to distal and is often first evident in muscles around the shoulder, trunk, and pelvic girdles, with patterns of muscle involvement specific and unique to each type of MD [1, 13, 15–18, 31, 33, 34]. As weakness increases, compensatory alterations are made in posture and movement to mechanically lock joints and substitute for lack of adequate muscle strength [11, 14, 19, 30, 31, 35]. The substitutions are effective in maximizing function but eventually lead to contracture and deformity that contribute to increasing weakness and disability [36, 37]. In addition to weakness that occurs due to actual muscle degeneration, weakness may also seem to "progress" in proportion to growth, as has also been described in other disorders characterized by weakness [38, 39]. The compromising impact and effect of gravity increases in magnitude with increased size as the muscles are less able to cope with an increase in mass, and during periods of rapid growth in which contracture can progress more rapidly.

Effective intervention is that which is focused on breaking this self-perpetuating cycle of events whenever possible so that strength can be maximally maintained, contracture and deformity can be minimized, and compensations can be used to maximize function without leading to increases in disability [14, 19].

The key to management of most neuromuscular diseases is in their predictability [1]. Muscle weakness progresses in specific and well-known orders and patterns [1, 13, 30, 31, 40–43]. Predictable compensations are used to cope with this increasing weakness [1, 33, 34, 44–46]. Specific muscle tightness, contracture, and deformity can result and occurs in predictable sequences without intervention [5, 6, 36, 40, 46] (Table 8.1). This predictability is a double-edged sword. On the one hand, the predictability is evidence of a progression that cannot yet be stopped. On the other hand, knowledge of the predictable progression empowers the multidisciplinary team, and the family, to plan ahead and intervene with prospective, preventative, anticipatory management. Many of the devastating secondary effects of the intrinsic myopathic process can be minimized with comprehensive, ongoing, anticipatory, and preventative management that maintains the highest possible quality of life despite disease progression [6, 55]. Multidisciplinary guidelines supporting this approach are available for increasing numbers of neuromuscular disorders [5, 6, 56, 57].

## Physical Therapy Assessment

Assessment must be ongoing and comprehensive so that intervention can be timely and anticipatory [6, 37]. Specific areas of weakness, tightness, and compensation should be identified in order to allow intervention that optimizes and protects muscle integrity and function, prevents contracture and deformity, and provides for effective adaptive functioning and participation to the greatest extent possible [6]. Assessment and intervention should occur across the ICF (the World Health Organization International Classification of Function [58]) and across the lifespan [5, 6, 55, 59] and should include impairment level measures, functional measures, and measures of participation, while considering the context and environmental factors of the individual [60]. Assessment and management of musculoskeletal and cardiorespiratory involvement and function requires a multidisciplinary team [5, 6] (Table 8.2).

## Physical Therapy Intervention

### Prevention of Contracture and Deformity

With weakness and compensation there may be no way to eliminate a compensatory pattern of movement without eliminating the function it serves, but it is important to try to find compensations that pose less of a risk of contracture and deformity and to try to avoid development of the contractures that contribute to the self-perpetuating evolution of weakness/contracture/functional loss [6, 14, 30, 31, 35]. The effects of chronic positioning, the unopposed influence of gravity, and imbalanced muscle

**Table 8.1** Patterns of skeletal muscle weakness, compensation, and resultant risk of secondary contracture and deformity in representative diagnoses: Duchenne/Becker Muscular Dystrophy (DMD/BMD), Facioscapulohumeral muscular dystrophy (FSHD) and Emery-Dreifuss Muscular Dystrophy (EDMD) [2, 13, 19, 24, 30, 31, 47–50]

DMD/BMD [2, 3, 6, 19, 30, 31, 33, 44] DMD/BMD weakness, as detailed in Chapter 4, tends to be symmetrical

| Characteristic weakness (early stage) | Characteristic compensations/posture/patterns of movement (early stage) | Tightness (early stage) |
|---|---|---|
| – Hip extensors (*gluteus maximus*)<br>– Ankle dorsiflexors (*anterior tibialis*)<br>– Hip abductors (*gluteus medius*)<br>– Hip adductors<br>– Abdominals<br>– Neck flexors (*sternocleidomastoid*)<br>– Shoulder depressors and extensors (*lower trap/latissimus*)<br>– Shoulder abductors (*deltoids*)<br>– Elbow extensors (*triceps*) | – Increased lumbar lordosis (posterior trunk lean) to keep force line behind hip joint (initially see *less* anterior pelvic tilt as hyperextension at hip joint in stance as long as quadriceps are strong enough to counteract moment into knee flexion)<br>– Lack of heelstrike<br>– Increased hip flexion during swing to clear foot<br>– Foot may be pronated and everted<br>– May see "hip waddling gait" as do not get adequate forward weight shift<br>– Increased UE abduction and lateral trunk sway<br>– Cadence decreases<br>– Gower's maneuver<br>– Neck and UE weakness not usually noticeable functionally but apparent with testing | May see emerging tightness in:<br>– Plantarflexors<br>– Hip flexors<br>– Iliotibial bands |
| Characteristic weakness (middle stage) | Characteristic compensations/posture/patterns of movement (middle stage) | Tightness (middle stage) |
| – Weakness progresses in muscles listed above<br>– Quadriceps weakness = key to gait deterioration<br>– Ankle everters (peroneals) | – Must get line of gravity simultaneously in front of knee joint and behind hip joint—uses:<br>  • Anterior pelvic tilt<br>  • Diminished hip extension in stance<br>  • Base of support widens:<br>  • Balance<br>  • Increased ankle plantarflexion and equinus positioning—to give torque that opposes knee flexion<br>– Begin to see increased falling<br>– Also get inversion with posterior tibialis relatively stronger—leads to unstable subtalar joint and more falling due to "twisting of the ankle"—although most falling is due to weakness in quadriceps and "knee buckling" | **Tightness** develops in:<br>– Iliotibial band and tensor fascia lata<br>– Hip flexors<br>– Hamstrings<br>– Gastrocsoleus<br>– Posterior tibialis<br>– **Important:** two-joint muscles get tight first |

| DMD/BMD [2, 3, 6, 19, 30, 31, 33, 44] DMD/BMD weakness, as detailed in Chapter 4, tends to be symmetrical | | |
| --- | --- | --- |
| *Characteristic weakness (later stage)* | *Characteristic compensations/posture/patterns of movement (later stages)* | *Tightness (later stages)* |
| – Weakness continues to progress in muscles listed above and becomes profound | – Prior to loss of ambulation, most compensations are used to maintain an upright posture and facilitate ambulation | – Accelerated development of LE contractures |
| – UE weakness becomes more significant functionally and is imbalanced: | – After loss of ambulation, compensatory movements are primarily used to: | – Beginning development of UE contractures |
| – Elbow extension weaker than flexion | • Achieve support and stability in sitting | – Tightness into elbow flexion and pronation |
| – Forearm supination weaker than pronation | • Assist UE function | – Tightness in wrist and finger flexors +/or extensors, lumbricals |
| – Wrist and finger extension weaker than flexion | – Compensatory movements include: | – Cervical spinal extensors and rotators |
| – Neck extensors, hamstrings, posterior tibialis are relatively spared until quite late in the disease | • Leaning for stability | *Scoliosis: the development of scoliosis is a major complication of the late or non-ambulatory stage, with natural history changing (decreasing) with steroids |
| – Distal hand function is relatively preserved, at least in long flexors but may be functionally compromised by lack of proximal stability and/or scoliosis requiring use of hands for sitting stability | • Contralateral trunk leaning during UE function to substitute for shoulder girdle weakness in arm lifting (deltoid weakness in abduction) | |
| | • Backward leaning/lurching to compensate for deltoid weakness in forward flexion and biceps weakness in elbow flexion | |
| | – Leading with head (especially using neck extensors) to shift weight and compensate for weak trunk musculature | |
| | – Using mouth to grab fingers and move arm to substitute for proximal UE musculature | |
| | – Pivoting forearm on elbow to substitute for elbow flexors | |

(continued)

**Table 8.1** (continued)

**FSHD** [4, 13, 47, 48, 51] FSHD clinical presentation much more variable than other diagnoses, as detailed in Chapter 3, with asymmetrical weakness not necessarily related to handedness

| Characteristic/possible weakness | Functional impact/compensation | Tightness/pain |
|---|---|---|
| – Facial muscles:<br>  Orbicularis oculi<br>  Orbicularis oris<br>  Zygomaticus<br>– Scapular muscles:<br>  Serratus anterior<br>  Middle and lower trapezius<br>– Horizontal abductor<br>– Pectoralis major<br>– Humeral muscles: (biceps brachii)<br>– Abdominal weakness—lower weaker than upper (Beevor sign)<br>– Hip extensors<br>– Knee flexors<br>– Anterior tibialis | – Scapular winging<br>– Compensatory use of momentum and distal strength to move arms<br>– Difficult closing eyes<br>– Difficulty pursing lips, drinking with straw, whistling<br>– Decreased ability to show facial expressiveness<br>– Anterior pelvic tilt<br>– Lumbar lordosis<br>– Foot drop<br>– Spinal asymmetry—with risk of scoliosis and tendency towards rigid spine in some | **Tightness** can develop in:<br>– Spinal musculature<br>– Neck musculature<br>– Hip flexors<br>– Plantarflexors<br>– Shoulder girdle musculature<br>**Scoliosis** is a risk as well as excessive spinal extension and sever lumbar lordosis<br>**Muscle pain** can be a prominent feature |

**EDMD** [52–54] Contractures are present early in relation to weakness, as detailed in Chapter 5, with less correlation to cycles of weakness and compensation

| Characteristic weakness | Compensatory/resultant posture | Tightness |
|---|---|---|
| – Slowly progressive muscle weakness in humero-peroneal pattern:<br>  • Initially proximal in upper extremities<br>  • Initially distal in lower extremities<br>  • Progresses to proximal limb-girdle pattern including vastii muscles, hamstrings, and adductors<br>– Selective early relative sparing of lateral gastrocnemius, and longer sparing of rectus femoris in EDMD2 | – Posture of increasing spinal extension, elbow flexion, plantarflexion<br>– Lateral trunk lean during ambulation<br>– Use of compensatory support mechanisms to maintain head control<br>– Use of compensatory mechanisms and momentum to optimize hand use | – Early contracture of:<br>  • Elbow flexors<br>  • Cervical spinal extensors<br>  • Plantarflexors<br>– Eventual tightness throughout spinal extensors at all levels |

**Table 8.2** Assessment tools across the ICF

| Impairment | Function | Disability measures | Quality of life/participation/activity | Person reported outcomes |
|---|---|---|---|---|
| – Passive ranges of motion and measures of muscle extensibility | Upper and lower extremity functional scales [13, 44, 61] | – PEDI (pediatric evaluation of disability index) [62] | – Peds QL [63] | – Fatigue scales [64–66] |
| – Identification of risks of tightness, contracture, and deformity | Timed functional tests [67, 68] | – Functional independence measure (FIM, WeeFIM) [69, 70] | – PODCI [71–76] | – Rate of perceived exertion [77–79] |
| – Muscle strength testing [80, 81]<br>• Manual muscle testing<br>• Dynamometry<br>• Computerized quantitative muscle assessment | GSGC (gait, stairs, Gowers, chair) [82, 83]<br>North Star Ambulatory Assessment [88–93]<br>Motor function measure (MFM) [95]<br>Modified Hammersmith functional motor scale and extend [98, 99]<br>Quick motor function test (QMFT) [100]<br>Egan klassification (EK) [103]<br>Alberta infant motor scales [104]<br>Gross motor function measure (GMFM) [105]<br>Peabody developmental motor scales-2 [106]<br>Bruininks-Oseretsky test of motor proficiency-2 (BOT-2) [107]<br>PUL [108]<br>Endurance:<br>  6 min walk test [109]<br>Observational gait analysis and kinematic analysis of movement, function, and compensatory patterns of movement | – Rotterdam handicap scale [84] | – Canadian occupational performance measure (COPM) [85, 86]<br>– Child Health Questionnaire [94]<br>– Activities scale for kids (ASK) [96, 97]<br>– Activity monitors [101, 102] | – Borg dyspnea scale [78, 87] |

aPain should be reported using age-appropriate pain scales [110–118] activity around joints contribute to the development of hypoextensibility (tightness) and contracture [2, 6, 11, 30, 35, 119]. Positioning for function and for management of the musculoskeletal system should be offered [6, 21, 23, 120–122].

*Stretching*: Prevention/minimization of contracture requires sufficient daily elongation of musculature and daily movement through more complete ranges of motion than the individual with MD typically uses actively and independently [1, 2, 6, 11, 21, 36, 44, 45, 119, 123]; these may be achieved through preventative stretching and varied positioning, facilitation of movement and position changes, use of therapeutic interventions including passive and active elongation, daily range of motion/stretching, the appropriate use of orthotic intervention, splinting, serial casting, power positioning components on mobility devices, participation in aquatics and cycling/assisted cycling and other forms of submaximal active movement and participation, and the use of adaptive equipment for positioning and prolonged passive elongation including the use of standers and stand-and-drive mobility devices [5, 6, 11, 19, 21, 23, 24, 37, 44, 45, 55, 119, 123–127]. A stretching program should begin early in the course of the disease and is more effective and more easily established as part of the daily routine if it is begun before muscle tightness/contracture is established and before stretching is uncomfortable. A preventative stretching program should address structures known to be at risk for tightness based on natural history of the specific diagnosis, as well as any structures identified by individual assessment to be at risk for contracture [6]. Direct and skilled physical therapy techniques of muscle elongation, joint mobilization, gentle manual traction, and use of modalities and other manual therapy techniques to increase joint mobility and muscle elongation should be included as appropriate for individual patients based on recommendations after individual physical therapy evaluation [128] (Table 8.3).

*Orthotic intervention/adaptive equipment*: Orthotic intervention may be recommended for function and/or for assistance in management of the musculoskeletal system and may include consideration of many different choices, configurations, and materials, for upper and lower extremities, trunk, and neck. Lower extremity orthotic intervention may include consideration of ankle–foot orthoses (AFOs or "short leg orthoses"), knee–ankle–foot orthoses (KAFOs or "long leg braces"), knee extension splints, inframalleolar orthoses ("foot orthoses"), or other types and configurations of orthoses, with control of varying degrees of freedom depending on specific diagnosis and individual assessment [6, 21, 23, 123, 129]. Upper extremity splinting, orthotic intervention, and support may include splinting for stretching or support of function [130] and is increasingly including exploration of exoskeletons and robotics to increase functional use of hands in the presence of proximal weakness [131, 132].

Use of lower extremity orthotic intervention and adaptive equipment for *function* during walking typically depends upon the distribution of weakness and the required use of compensatory patterns of movement for function. In the presence of relatively greater proximal weakness in individuals who are independently ambulatory, such as in Duchenne muscular dystrophy (DMD), the use of AFOs during walking is not typically recommended. This is because AFOs tend to compromise ambulation by

**Table 8.3** Muscles/joints/tissue commonly at risk for tightness in MDs (specifics depend on specific diagnosis)[a]

| Lower extremities | Upper extremities | Spine |
|---|---|---|
| *Muscles/soft tissue*: | *Muscles/soft tissue*: | Spinal extensors (including cervical) |
| Hip flexors | Shoulder musculature | Intercostals |
| Iliotibial bands | Elbow flexors | Risk of: |
| Hamstrings | Forearm pronators | – Scoliosis |
| Plantarflexors, especially gastrocnemius | Wrist and finger flexors and/or extensors | – Excessive kyphosis |
| Posterior tibialis | Lumbricals | – Excessive lordosis |
| Plantar fascia | | – Pelvic asymmetries and mal-alignment |
| Two joint muscles get tight first | Two joint muscles get tight first | Excessive anterior pelvic tilt |
| *Joints—risk of contracture into*: | *Joints—risk of contracture into*: | Excessive posterior pelvic tilt |
| Hip flexion | Elbow flexion | Lateral pelvic tilt |
| Knee flexion | Wrist flexion (or extension) | Horizontal pelvic rotation |
| Ankle plantarflexion | Flexion at isolated finger joints (PIP, DIP) Extension at isolated finger joints (PIP, DIP) | |

[a]Any muscles, joints, soft tissue or structures may be at risk for tightness, contracture, deformity based on individual assessment of typical/chronic posture, function, muscle imbalance, compensatory patterns of movement, and the influence of gravity

limiting the use of compensations needed for walking, such as toe-walking or intermittent toe-walking, may compromise proximal compensations needed to keep the line of gravity behind the hip and in front of the knee to maintain ambulation, and may make it more difficult to get up from the floor, with the added weight of AFOs further compromising function [6, 129]. In other types of MD characterized by relatively greater distal than proximal weakness, or in which more global weakness is present, such as in some types of congenital myopathy, AFOs may assist in providing distal stability. This can be beneficial during standing and/or ambulation as long as AFOs are lightweight enough and offer optimal support without unnecessarily compromising function or movement that is necessary for function. Newer, ultra-lightweight carbon fiber AFOs used in conjunction with lower profile orthotic intervention at the foot and ankle may offer lightweight support without compromising function in those with greater distal than proximal weakness. This can potentially offer dorsiflexion assist during swing to prevent "foot drop" and "steppage gait" and potentially provide some floor-reaction support of knee extension during stance and may decrease fatigue. Ankle height or supramalleolar orthoses (SMOs) are not typically helpful because they add weight that challenges active dorsiflexion (typically weak in MDs) without adding dorsiflexion assist. However, these could be considered in the rare situation in which weakness is extremely mild, with good strength in anterior tibialis, but with poor medial–lateral alignment that requires more support than an inframalleolar orthosis. KAFOs may be useful in children with greater weakness throughout lower extremities in the absence of the ability to support weight-bearing independently. This approach has been shown to extend walking for several years in some individuals with DMD when independent walking becomes too difficult because of inability to support weight through lower extremities without support and/or inability to maintain biomechanical positioning to mechanically lock joints in support of weight-bearing and ambulation [46, 55, 121, 133–136]. Braced ambulation with KAFOs may be therapeutic rather than functional across settings [46] and is most often used in combination with motorized mobility for functional, safe, independent mobility in settings in which braced ambulation is not functional or does not allow optimal participation.

Use of lower extremity orthotic intervention and adaptive equipment for *musculoskeletal management* (to prevent contracture and deformity) may include the use of AFOs [6, 21, 123], KAFOs [23, 55, 133], thigh binders, splints, serial casting [126, 127], or other positioning devices at night [21] or in the evening or during any portions of the day when they will not unduly interfere with function [6]. The use of AFOs at night has been shown to minimize the progression of plantarflexion contractures [21] and is recommended if tolerated. AFOs used at night need to be comfortable and should be custom molded and lightweight enough not to unduly restrict bed mobility. A bed or foot tent can hold the blanket up off of the feet to avoid the feet getting tangled in the sheets. Adjustable angle orthoses can sometimes be used to provide differing amounts of stretch at different times of the day, or gradually increasing elongation for comfort. The use of ankle height or SMOs may be helpful for those using a wheelchair full time, in order to assist in maintaining optimal medial–lateral alignment if the footplate of the chair can be successfully used to limit excessive plantarflexion. The number of hours per day that a muscle is in a lengthened vs. shortened position will influence the development or prevention of contracture. Standard recommendations for prevention of progressive contracture support the maintenance of a lengthened position for six of every 24 h [137]. The use of standers and stand-and-drive motorized mobility devices is recommended for providing prolonged passive elongation into simultaneous hip and knee extension in an upright weight-bearing for optimizing and maintaining joint range of motion, providing muscle elongation over multiple joints, and optimizing bone integrity, if tolerated [20, 55, 133, 134, 138, 139].

*Prevention/minimization of spinal deformity* typically involves: promotion of symmetry through the vertebral column and pelvis; support of appropriate amounts of extension and flexion at specific levels of the vertebral column; maintenance of flexibility; support of optimal posture; and minimization of the asymmetrical deforming forces of compensatory patterns of movements used for function (in most neuromuscular disorders) or intrinsic to diagnosis (such as in FSH). The progression of spinal deformity in neuromuscular disorders has been well studied, and understanding of the individual pathokinesiology in each diagnosis and detailed assessment and management of the interaction between components in each individual are critical. The development and progression of scoliosis has been most extensively studied in DMD, which can be used as a model to understand the pathokinesiology, and can inform conservative treatment. The natural history of scoliosis is changing with the use of steroids in DMD, with scoliosis appearing later, and with less devastating progression [140].

*Scoliosis in ambulatory individuals* with DMD has been studied [141, 142] and is characterized by a flexible, functional scoliosis related to asymmetrical lower extremity position/contracture, pelvic obliquity, asymmetrical realignment of shoulders, head, and upper extremities [35, 143, 144]. Fixed spinal asymmetry is typically minimized spontaneously in ambulatory individuals by prolonged, protective spinal hyperextension and locking of posterior intervertebral facet joints at lumbar and lumbosacral levels, and alternating torso shift and lateral trunk elongation [11, 35, 145].

Historically, prolongation of ambulation by management of lower extremity contracture and the use of long leg braces appeared to slow the development of scoliosis in some [146], likely via prolongation of protective spinal hyperextension maybe through the adolescent growth spurt, and continued torso shift and lateral trunk elongation over symmetrical lower extremities [35, 145, 147, 148]. Factors that have appeared to influence whether or not scoliosis appears prior to final loss of ambulation included: the age at which walking ceases; intervention used or not used to prolong ambulation; and final gait pattern [146].

It has generally been agreed that spinal curves during the ambulatory period are not usually "fixed" (i.e., rigid or inflexible), are functionally necessary for ambulation, and cannot be corrected without risking the loss of ambulation [35]. Attempts should be made, therefore, to minimize long-term effects of asymmetry with stretching, positioning, etc., while allowing compensations necessary for function. In individuals with intrinsic asymmetry of weakness, as has been identified in FSH, and extreme anterior pelvic tilt and lumbar lordosis, the use of a soft corset during ambulation may provide support that decreases pain and fatigue during ambulation without compromising compensations to the extent that ambulation is compromised.

*Scoliosis in non-ambulatory individuals*: Scoliosis as a significant problem in DMD and other neuromuscular disorders typically either begins or develops more rapidly as ambulation is lost and full time use of a wheelchair begins [35, 149]. It is one of the most serious and disabling complications of many neuromuscular disorders and has been studied extensively in DMD, with the understanding of the principles of progression and treatment gained in DMD useful in the management of all neuromuscular scoliosis [150]. Neuromuscular scoliosis can progress to a level of incapacitating severity that compromises pulmonary function, sitting ability, upper extremity function, comfort, and cosmetic integrity [11, 35]. The progression of scoliosis is variable, however, and final deformity ranges from mild in some individuals to severe in others [150]. The significance of the variability is in the opportunity it offers for effecting change and for making use of intervention that may prevent or minimize the development of scoliosis. Attempts at successful management must be based on a comprehensive understanding of the factors that contribute to the development of scoliosis. Aggressive conservative management must be coordinated with consideration of surgical options in order to prevent the catastrophic progression to severe deformity in all individuals with MDs.

Factors that contribute to the development of scoliosis can be divided into those factors that make the spine vulnerable and those factors that initiate asymmetry [151].

**Factors That Make the Spine Vulnerable [151]:**
- *Severe symmetrical weakness in trunk musculature* [150, 152]

  - Decreases spinal support and stability.
  - Without external support, the spine is vulnerable to external forces it cannot oppose.

- *Rapid vertebral growth during adolescent growth spurt* [152, 153]

  - Often coincides with, or follows, the loss of ambulation.
  - Increases vulnerability to potentially deforming forces (the musculoskeletal system is known to be more vulnerable to any deforming force during periods of rapid growth).

- *Loss of protective spinal hyperextension* [11, 19, 154, 155]

  - Spinal hyperextension is decreased or eliminated when individuals begin to sit full time [156].
  - Posterior intervertebral facet joints are unlocked and allow more lateral flexion (bending) and rotation [19, 150, 156].
  - Stretching of posterior spinal ligaments increases with kyphosis [150].
  - Can be exacerbated by posterior pelvic tilt caused by tight hamstrings and lower extremity alignment in sitting.

**Asymmetrical forces imposed** on the symmetrically weak and vulnerable spine [151]:
- *Compensatory movement patterns* used:

  - *For stability*—Tend to lean on one arm of the wheelchair, may lean forward also—tends to push that shoulder up.
  - *For upper extremity (UE) function*—Use lateral trunk flexion towards the contralateral (opposite) side when elevating or abducting one upper extremity, in order to substitute for weak shoulder muscles, with persistent leaning towards the non-dominant side, may contribute to development of a curve with convexity towards the side of dominance [152, 157].

- *Pelvic position*:

  - *Posterior pelvic tilt* [11, 150]

    ○ Can further exacerbate an asymmetrical loss of spinal hyperextension by asymmetrically tightness in hamstrings [150]

  - *Pelvic obliquity* (lateral pelvic tilt) [11, 35, 150]
  - *Pelvic rotation* (in horizontal plane) [150]

    ○ Pelvic rotation and obliquity can be present in sitting from:

      ▪ *Preexisting asymmetry of soft tissue contracture* around hips and pelvis [35] (for example: hip flexors, iliotibial bands)

- *Asymmetrical pelvic position* in the absence of asymmetrical contracture, from [11, 150]
    - Sling seat
    - Poorly fitting wheelchair
    - Any unstable sitting surface
  - *Lower extremity position* [30, 35]
    - *Hips* can have a direct effect on pelvis, then spine, as described above:
      - Asymmetrical hip flexor and/or iliotibial band tightness or contracture
      - Tight hamstrings leading to posterior pelvic tilt and kyphosis
    - *Foot/ankle* asymmetrical contracture into equinovarus from unopposed posterior tibialis and gastrocsoleus—tighter side pushes pelvis back into ipsilateral posterior horizontal pelvic rotation.

The deforming force of **gravity** on the vertebral column increases in the presence of asymmetrical spinal-pelvic alignment that compromises the simple mechanical ability of the vertebral column to withstand the force of gravity. In addition, the resultant unequal distribution of weight on epiphyseal growth plates increases the potential for an initial flexible scoliosis to become structural.

**Interaction Between Factors**

- Symmetrically weak and vulnerable spine is present in all individuals with DMD when ambulation ceases.
- Particular vulnerability is present in those who lose protective spinal hyperextension. This is the initiating factor that is imposed upon the spine with the potential to cause asymmetry and progressive scoliosis. It may include any one of previously described factors and may be different in each person.
- Once asymmetry is initiated, secondary asymmetries are established and spinal deformities can progress in a self-perpetuating circle of weakness, compensation, and contracture.

Management of the spine must be anticipatory and preventative with consideration across the continuum of intervention options, including stretching, positioning, external support, and surgical options, with coordination between the multidisciplinary team. The use and timing of anticipatory and preventative conservative measures is coordinated with ongoing assessment regarding the potential need for surgical stabilization to manage curves that progress in spite of conservative measures. Care must be taken to coordinate with the rest of the team, with particular coordination between PT, orthopedics, pulmonary medicine, and cardiology, as conservative measures are employed. This helps ensure that the window of opportunity for surgical spinal stabilization (which is dependent on the interaction between pulmonary, respiratory, and cardiology status) is not missed, if the individual will need surgical stabilization at some point (see Chapter 9).

Intervention described in the literature has included prolongation of ambulation, external support including bracing, specialized seating systems, wheelchair modifications, promotion of upper extremity symmetry, control of lower extremity position, and spinal surgery. Bracing of the spine in individuals with DMD has historically not been tolerated or successful but may have a role in other diagnoses and situations, especially in younger children with myopathies characterized by more profound trunk weakness at earlier ages. Orthotic intervention may include supportive garments, corsets, or spine jackets in younger children with some types of MD in order to support more vertical, symmetrical, and extended spinal alignment and more stable posture and stability in upright. Such interventions may assist in maintaining spinal symmetry, or providing some support which may be beneficial in ambulatory individuals in whom some support is helpful but must avoid excessive restriction of movement that may limit compensatory movement required for ambulation [158–160].

Optimal support and positioning in seating systems is critical in musculoskeletal management of the spine and extremities and must include maintenance of midline, symmetrical pelvic position with prevention of lateral pelvic tilt, horizontal pelvic rotation, and excessive anterior or posterior pelvic tilt; maintenance of a midline erect spine, and support of a symmetrical midline head position. Typical recommendations include: a solid seat and back; rigid lateral trunk supports; hip guides; adductors; a head rest and adequate upper extremity and foot and leg support; with power positioning components for power tilt, power recline, separately elevating power elevating leg rests, power adjustable seat height, and power standing [6]. Seating system components are needed for support for function, prevention of progressive contracture and deformity, and maintenance of skin integrity. Power positioning components are needed for function, for independent position change for prevention of contracture and deformity, for support of adequate frequency and duration of weight-bearing throughout the day, and for provision of independent weight shift and pressure relief throughout the day that is adequate to maintain skin integrity.

Physical therapy management of the spine in the individual with MD must involve ongoing evaluation and intervention. Ongoing evaluation must attend to the asymmetrical forces acting on the vulnerable spine and should include assessment of:

- Pelvic position
- Spinal alignment including

  - Medial–lateral alignment
  - Rotational tendencies
  - Amount of extension
  - Symmetry vs. asymmetry

- Lower extremity position and its effect on the spine
- Compensatory movement patterns and positioning

**Goals of PT Management of the Spine**
- Maintain ambulation and standing as long as possible
- Promote spinal extension in sitting except in diagnoses or situations characterized by excessive extension, such as EDMD or in rigid spine syndromes [145]

- Maintain maximal symmetry of positioning in wheelchair
- Limit use of compensatory movement patterns that lead to deformity
- Provide for UE function with symmetry
- Maintain flexibility

**Suggestions for Wheelchair Management**
- **Wheelchair support/positioning**—the individual's chair should fit well and provide support that achieves:
- *Sitting position* characterized by:

  - A level pelvis without obliquity or rotation
  - A straight, erect, midline spinal position
  - Elimination of kyphosis and encouragement of extension except in diagnoses or situations characterized by excessive extension, such as EDMD or in rigid spine syndromes
  - Symmetrical LE position with good foot placement (not too much plantarvarus) and without hip abduction

- *Sufficient trunk support* so that asymmetrical leaning is not necessary for maintenance of an upright position
- *Control of asymmetrical movement patterns*
- Specific recommendations for *wheelchair seating system components* include:

  - Solid seat attached to frame of chair
  - Solid back attached to frame of chair
  - Pelvic control in all planes:

    ◦ Hip control blocks (hip guides)
    ◦ Seat belt appropriately located and/or adapted
    ◦ subASIS bar?

  - *Knee pads* to control abduction (adductor pads)
  - *Planar, rigid, lateral trunk supports*—appropriately located and *strong* enough to:

    ◦ Prevent the need to lean laterally for stability
    ◦ Stop compensatory lean for UE function

  - *Control of lower extremity position*—might include:

    ◦ Foot plate appropriately located and angled
    ◦ Ankle straps
    ◦ Padded footrests or foot cradles
    ◦ AFO's
    ◦ Surgical correction of ankle–foot deformity

  - *Arm rests* appropriately located to encourage spinal extension rather than kyphosis
  - *Chest strap* (in older individual) in order to provide additional support that centers trunk and allows leaning into lordosis [161]

  – *Lumbar roll* as appropriate to encourage spinal extension
  – *Head support* (customized as needed)

• Power tilt-in-space, power recline, with separately elevating power elevating
  leg rests, for

  – Changes in position, maintenance of skin integrity
  – Opening up of hip and knee angles to assist in minimizing the development
    of contractures

• Power standing
• Power seat elevation (power adjustable seat height)

## Control of Asymmetrical Compensatory Movement Patterns

• Evaluate during **all** functional activities (wheelchair driving or propulsion,
  writing, eating)
• **Stop compensatory lean**!
• Provide for function with symmetry—might include:
  – Relocation of wheelchair controls (joystick)

    ◦ Closer to hand on wheelchair arm to prevent need for reaching
    ◦ Use of non-dominant hand?
    ◦ Alternate sides periodically?
    ◦ Central location? (but this can compromise stability and increase need
      for leaning)

  – Raised desk/tray/table height—works very well to allow pivoting of arm
    on elbow
  – Overhead sling
  – Balanced forearm orthoses
  – Robotic/exoskeleton forearm support
  – Other adaptive equipment

• **Standing**—to assist in control of LE contracture and to encourage spinal
  extension as well as offering more general physiological benefits and increased
  function
• **Maintaining flexibility**

  – Elongation in prone, supine, or sidelying to maintain symmetrical lateral
    elongation and flexibility
  – Maximally preventing contractures in lower extremities

• **Parent/child education**

  – Educate individual and caretakers about symmetry vs. asymmetry and
    goals of spinal management as described above
  – Have individual monitor symmetry vs. asymmetry with visual feedback at
    mirror periodically, and when making changes in support or positioning to
    establish accurate "feel" of symmetry

It is important to stop and consciously reassess postural alignment at regular intervals — even as frequently every three months in addition to daily awareness.

The above spinal management plan outlines conservative measures that can be used in an attempt to prevent the progression of scoliosis in individuals with DMD. Close coordination with the rest of the medical team is important in identification of those individuals in whom conservative measures are not working so that more aggressive means, such as surgery, can be used for spinal management.

Spinal surgery is discussed in detail elsewhere (see Chapter 9).

## Optimizing strength

Concern about whether or not strengthening activities hasten the progression of weakness in dystrophic muscles are longstanding and exist for many reasons, yet precise knowledge regarding what types of muscle activity may be detrimental or beneficial is limited [22, 172–187]. A certain amount of muscle activity has been assumed to be beneficial in preventing disuse atrophy, maintaining residual strength, providing or maintaining a potential trophic influence of active movement on muscle, and maintaining functional status and flexibility [174, 182, 183, 187]. Overwork weakness, however, should be avoided, as should exercise-induced damage [182, 183]. Eccentric muscle activity and maximal resistive exercise are believed to be detrimental to fragile muscles and should be avoided [183]. Submaximal aerobic exercise within the limits of pain and fatigue is generally supported, balanced by the use of energy conservation techniques for support of function and participation [174, 182, 183, 187] with respiratory muscle training supported by some with similar caution about overexertion [167, 188–192].

## Managing/minimizing pain

This often involves assessment and correction of posture; assessment and correction of abnormal or excessive pressure imposed by abnormal posture, immobility, and abnormal weight-bearing with decreased ability to change positions; muscle tightness and/or over-lengthening, imbalanced muscle activity, and functional compensations; patterns and presence of overuse; fatigue; with consideration of other factors such as fracture and cardiac etiology important in settings of acute, new onset, or changing pain [193]. The use of energy conservation techniques and analysis of ergonomics during function are important in prevention and reduction of pain, as is the provision of appropriate adaptive equipment to support function, movement, position change, and pressure relieving surfaces for sitting and sleeping. More direct treatment for relief of pain should be coordinated by the multidisciplinary team and may include PT interventions using modalities of heat, cold, TENS, and massage [47].

**Respiratory Management [162–164]**

- Comprehensive evaluation and management by pulmonary medicine specialists is recommended [162, 163, 165, 166]
- Respiratory function can be compromised by a number of factors:

  – Progressive muscle weakness interacts with spinal/thoracic deformity to result in severe decline in pulmonary function.
  – Intrinsic lung disease is *not* typically present.

- Involvement typically includes:

**Less effective breathing due to muscle weakness**

- Weakness may present and progress in respiratory muscles including diaphragm, intercostal muscles, abdominal muscles, and accessory muscles of respiration such as neck flexors, depending on the specific diagnosis.
- A diaphragmatic pattern of breathing may be used with very little intercostal activity. This restricted pattern of breathing and increasing muscle weakness leads to an inability to expand and compress the lungs fully.
- Total lung capacity, vital capacity, and forced inspiratory and expiratory abilities decrease and residual volume increases.
- Progression:

Shallow breathing

↓

More rapid breathing (to get rid of $CO_2$)

↓

Less chest or lung volume/expansion

↓

Decreased breathing volume

- **Decreased lung expansion**: leads to little areas of collapse of lung tissue (i.e., atelectasis vulnerable to infection).
- **Decreased coughing ability**: due to weakness in abdominals and muscles of forced expiration as well as decreased ability to take a deep breath just before coughing. This leads to retention of secretions.
- **Restricted thoracic mobility** and stiffening of the chest wall result from fibrous replacement of the muscles of the thoracic wall as well as from restricted patterns of breathing and decreased lung movement. This leads to further decrease in lung mobility and expansion. It may be accompanied by ankylosing of the joints.
- **Impact of spinal deformity** on respiratory status: Respiratory insufficiency compounded by scoliosis when present.
- **Goals of interventions**:

  – Maintain chest wall mobility
  – Maintain strength and endurance in respiratory muscles as much as possible, possibly with submaximal exercise, especially when young (and also by providing them with sufficient rest with non-invasive ventilation as needed) [167].

- Establish and maintain most efficient breathing pattern possible
- Establish good pulmonary hygiene
- Coordinate with pulmonary team
- Support appropriate use of noninvasive inspiratory and expiratory aids

- **Suggestions**:

  - Inspiratory exercises/segmental breathing

    - To strengthen diaphragm gently, as appropriate, depending on diagnosis
    - For lung expansion and chest wall mobility
    - For more efficient breathing

  - Swimming

    - Breath control
    - Breathing patterns
    - Endurance

  - Practice coughing and use of mechanical assistance (manual assistance, ambu-bag)
  - GPB—glossopharyngeal breathing
  - Airway clearance techniques with postural drainage as necessary, with use of percussion or oscillatory vest
  - Periodic review of pulmonary hygiene techniques for at home
  - Spinal program to attempt to avoid potential further compromise of respiratory system by scoliosis
  - Inspiratory muscle aids: for example, nocturnal or daytime non-invasive ventilatory support
  - Expiratory muscle aids: for example, mechanical insufflation–exsufflation (MIE)—Cough Assist™
  - Coordination with team for anticipatory management regarding potential tracheostomy if necessary.

## Cardiac [168]

Cardiac muscle can be affected by the dystrophic process and anticipatory, preventative, comprehensive evaluation and management by cardiology is recommended [168–171]. Myocardial fibrosis may occur, primarily involving the free wall of the left ventricle. Cardiac involvement may also be affected by respiratory status and by scoliosis that, if severe, can cause direct cardiac compression. Cardiac involvement is frequently progressive and may be eventually characterized by the ECG abnormalities, hypertrophic cardiomyopathy, and dilated cardiomyopathy [171].

Cardiac involvement across the spectrum of MDs may also include AV block, atrial paralysis, atrial fibrillation or flutter, ventricular arrhythmia, conduction defects, and reduced ejection fraction [171].

Cardiac involvement in Becker muscular dystrophy [171] is often out of proportion with skeletal muscle involvement, additionally taxed by increased level of gross motor activity, with cardiac transplantation a viable option in some cases. Emery Dreifuss muscular dystrophy (EDMD) is typically characterized by cardiac conduction defects [53]. Cardiac care of individuals in MDs is more anticipatory and preventative than in the past. With increased survival, pacemakers and defibrillators are beginning to be used for some individuals [169].

Carriers of DMD/BMD may have cardiac manifestations and should be assessed and followed [170].

## *Maintaining Function*

- At every age, and every stage, age-appropriate function, participation in all aspects of life in which the individual is interested, and maximal independence should be supported.
- The bottom line should always be—"can he/she keep up with his/her peers?"
- Technology is the key to freedom in many situations.

### Adaptive Equipment and Assistive Technology

- Mobility devices:
    - Manual, motorized, power assist, scooters
    - Custom seating
    - Power positioning components:
        ○ Power tilt
        ○ Power recline
        ○ Separately elevating power elevating leg rests
        ○ Powered seat elevation
        ○ Powered standing and powered stand and drive

- Cycles, power assist cycles
- Standers
- Power adjustable beds and pressure relieving mattresses
- Lifts and transfer devices, powered lift (including ceiling lifts, pivot lifts, stair lifts, powered patient lifts)
- Upper extremity supports (forearm supports, robotics elbow blocks to keep hand from sliding away from joystick)
- Mini-proportional joy sticks
- Computer access, infra-red environmental control, bluetooth, voice activation, eye gaze systems
- Internet access
- Environmental control units (infra-red and bluetooth)
- Prism glasses for reading in bed or with limited mobility in neck flexion
- Bidets

- Bath and shower chairs
- Respiratory equipment:
    - Cough assist
    - BiPAP and noninvasive ventilation
    - Vest

- Ramps, portable ramps, van lifts, vertical platform lifts
- Bathing and bathrooming equipment that fosters ease and independence
- Power operated beds
- Handheld devices (smart phones, tablets, etc.)
- Modified sports equipment

**Sports/Adapted Sports**

- Swimming, cycling, wheelchair/adapted sports, dance

# Conclusion

Remarkable advances and progress in research raise hopes for finding treatments and cures for many of the genetically determined neuromuscular disorders. If quality of life is the focus for all individuals as we wait for more specific treatment and cures, effective intervention can be offered in many areas by using continually updated skills and resources, ingenuity, and a comprehensive understanding of each neuromuscular disorder. Comprehensive, anticipatory physical therapy (PT) management of MD is based upon an understanding of the pathokinesiology of each type of MD, an understanding of the progression of the pathokinesiology over time, individual evaluation within the context of each individual's life and goals, and provision of consistent, anticipatory, preventative management across the lifespan in order to minimize the clinical and functional impact of the diagnosis and to optimize quality of life. Optimal management is important for each individual not only for the sake of each day that is experienced as we wait for a cure but also for protection of the future that unfolds for that individual, and in order to help individuals stay in the best possible condition to make use of cures as they are found.

# Helpful Websites

## *Information About Diagnoses*

http://www.parentprojectmd.org
http://www.mdausa.org/
http://www.mdausa.org/disease/40list.html (list of diagnoses covered by Muscular Dystrophy Association (MDA)

http://www.fsma.org/
http://www.ninds.nih.gov/disorders/charcot_marie_tooth/detail_charcot_marie_
 tooth.htm
http://www.pompe.org.uk/
http://www.amda-pompe.org/
http://www.pompe.com/healthcare/pc_eng_hc_main.asp
https://www.genetests.org/
http://www.emedicine.com/neuro/topic668.htm
http://curecmd.org/
http://www.childmuscleweakness.org/

## Adaptive Equipment/Assistive Technology/Orthotic Intervention

### Orthotic Intervention

http://www.dafo.com/

### Lifts, Bathing, and Bathrooming Equipment

http://www.arjo.com/
http://www.image-management.com/
http://www.surehands.com/
http://www.bfl-inc.com/index.php

### Respiratory Care
www.coughassistt70.respironics.com
http://www.thevest.com/

Oximeters: http://www.pulseoximeter.org/

### Car Seats for Fragile Infants

http://www.eztether.com/index.php/instructions/hope-car-bed

### Standers

http://www.easystand.com/
http://mulhollandinc.com/products/rocket/
http://www.permobil.com

### Wheelchairs/Mobility Devices

http://www.permobil.com
http://www.pridemobility.com/
http://www.dekaresearch.com/ibot.shtml
http://www.frankmobility.com/e-fix.php

### Cycling

http://www.exnflex.com/

## Other

http://www.portable-wheelchair-ramps.com/
http://www.ableplay.org/
http://accessiblelivingltd.com/portableramps.htm
http://www.aelseating.com/
http://www.easystand.com/
http://www.exnflex.com/
http://www.ezlock.net/
http://www.invacare.com/cgi-bin/imhqprd/index.jsp
http://www.kayeproducts.com/
http://www.adaptivemall.com/lectoilshowc.html
http://www.mulhollandinc.com/
http://www.ncatp.org/
http://www.portable-wheelchair-ramps.com/
http://www.pridemobility.com/
http://www.primeengineering.com/
http://www.quickie-wheelchairs.com/
http://www.rifton.com/index.htm
http://www.ezonpro.com/index.shtml
http://www.adaptivemall.com/tilslidrecba.html
http://www.duralife-usa.com/index.htm?group=5&content=2005
http://www.usatechguide.org/itemreview.php?itemid=846
http://www.permobilusa.com/templates/startpage.aspx?id=806
http://www.nadachair.com/
http://www.panthera.se/en/produkt_x.html
http://kinovarobotics.com/
http://www.pro-bed.com/
http://www.volker.co.uk/index.php

# References

1. Vignos PJ. Rehabilitation in progressive muscular dystrophy. New Haven: Licht; 1968.
2. Dubowitz V. Progressive muscular dystrophy: prevention of deformities. Clin Pediatr (Phila). 1964;12:323–8.
3. Dubowitz V. Muscle disorders in childhood. 2nd ed. London: Saunders; 1995.
4. Bushby KM, Pollitt C, Johnson MA, Rogers MT, Chinnery PF. Muscle pain as a prominent feature of facioscapulohumeral muscular dystrophy (FSHD): four illustrative case reports. Neuromuscul Disord. 1998;8(8):574–9.
5. Bushby K, Finkel R, Birnkrant DJ, et al. Diagnosis and management of Duchenne muscular dystrophy, part 1: diagnosis, and pharmacological and psychosocial management. Lancet Neurol. 2010;9(1):77–93.
6. Bushby K, Finkel R, Birnkrant DJ, et al. Diagnosis and management of Duchenne muscular dystrophy, part 2: implementation of multidisciplinary care. Lancet Neurol. 2010;9(2):177–89.
7. Bushby KM. The muscular dystrophies. Baillieres Clin Neurol. 1994;3(2):407–30.

8. Bushby KM, Gardner-Medwin D, Nicholson LV, et al. The clinical, genetic and dystrophin characteristics of Becker muscular dystrophy. II. Correlation of phenotype with genetic and protein abnormalities. J Neurol. 1993;240(2):105–12.

9. Bushby KM, Gardner-Medwin D. The clinical, genetic and dystrophin characteristics of Becker muscular dystrophy. I. Natural history. J Neurol. 1993;240(2):98–104.

10. Guglieri M, Straub V, Bushby K, Lochmuller H. Limb-girdle muscular dystrophies. Curr Opin Neurol. 2008;21(5):576–84.

11. Dubowitz V. Prevention of deformities. Isr J Med Sci. 1977;13(2):183–8.

12. Wang CH, Bonnemann CG, Rutkowski A, et al. Consensus statement on standard of care for congenital muscular dystrophies. J Child Neurol. 2010;25(12):1559–81.

13. Personius KE, Pandya S, King WM, Tawil R, McDermott MP. Facioscapulohumeral dystrophy natural history study: standardization of testing procedures and reliability of measurements. The FSH DY Group. Phys Ther. 1994;74(3):253–63.

14. Roy L, Gibson DA. Pseudohypertrophic muscular dystrophy and its surgical management: review of 30 patients. Can J Surg. 1970;13(1):13–21.

15. Kilmer DD, Abresch RT, McCrory MA, et al. Profiles of neuromuscular diseases. Facioscapulohumeral muscular dystrophy. Am J Phys Med Rehabil. 1995;74(5 Suppl):S131–9.

16. McDonald CM, Abresch RT, Carter GT, Fowler Jr WM, Johnson ER, Kilmer DD. Profiles of neuromuscular diseases. Becker's muscular dystrophy. Am J Phys Med Rehabil. 1995;74(5 Suppl):S93–103.

17. McDonald CM, Abresch RT, Carter GT, et al. Profiles of neuromuscular diseases. Duchenne muscular dystrophy. Am J Phys Med Rehabil. 1995;74(5 Suppl):S70–92.

18. McDonald CM, Johnson ER, Abresch RT, Carter GT, Fowler Jr WM, Kilmer DD. Profiles of neuromuscular diseases. Limb-girdle syndromes. Am J Phys Med Rehabil. 1995;74(5 Suppl):S117–30.

19. Fowler Jr WM. Rehabilitation management of muscular dystrophy and related disorders: II. Comprehensive care. Arch Phys Med Rehabil. 1982;63(7):322–8.

20. Miller G, Dunn N. An outline of the management and prognosis of Duchenne muscular dystrophy in Western Australia. Aust Paediatr J. 1982;18(4):277–82.

21. Scott OM, Hyde SA, Goddard C, Dubowitz V. Prevention of deformity in Duchenne muscular dystrophy. A prospective study of passive stretching and splintage. Physiotherapy. 1981;67(6):177–80.

22. Scott OM, Hyde SA, Goddard C, Jones R, Dubowitz V. Effect of exercise in Duchenne muscular dystrophy. Physiotherapy. 1981;67(6):174–6.

23. Hyde SA, Scott OM, Goddard CM, Dubowitz V. Prolongation of ambulation in Duchenne muscular dystrophy by appropriate orthoses. Physiotherapy. 1982;68(4):105–8.

24. Johnson ER, Fowler Jr WM, Lieberman JS. Contractures in neuromuscular disease. Arch Phys Med Rehabil. 1992;73(9):807–10.

25. Cherry DB. Review of physical therapy alternatives for reducing muscle contracture. Phys Ther. 1980;60(7):877–81.

26. Harris SE, Cherry DB. Childhood progressive muscular dystrophy and the role of physical therapy. Phys Ther. 1974;54(1):4–12.

27. Johnson LB, Florence JM, Abresch RT. Physical therapy evaluation and management in neuromuscular diseases. Phys Med Rehabil Clin N Am. 2012;23(3):633–51.

28. Stuberg WA. Muscular dystrophy and spinal muscular atrophy. In: Campbell SK, et al, editors. Physical therapy for children. St. Louis: Elsevier Saunders; 2012.

29. Gardner-Medwin D. Management of muscular dystrophy. Physiotherapy. 1977;63(2):46–51.

30. Siegel IM. Pathomechanics of stance in Duchenne muscular dystrophy. Arch Phys Med Rehabil. 1972;53(9):403–6.

31. Sutherland DH, Olshen R, Cooper L, et al. The pathomechanics of gait in Duchenne muscular dystrophy. Dev Med Child Neurol. 1981;23(1):3–22.

32. Hsu JD, Furumasu J. Gait and posture changes in the Duchenne muscular dystrophy child. Clin Orthop Relat Res. 1993;288:122–5.

33. Siegel IM, Weiss LA. Postural substitution in Duchenne's muscular dystrophy. JAMA. 1982;247(5):584.

34. Chyatte SB, Vignos Jr PJ, Watkins M. Early muscular dystrophy: differential patterns of weakness in Duchenne, limb-girdle and facioscapulohumeral types. Arch Phys Med Rehabil. 1966;47(8):499–503.
35. Siegel IM. Scoliosis in muscular dystrophy. Some comments about diagnosis, observations on prognosis, and suggestions for therapy. Clin Orthop Relat Res. 1973;93:235–8.
36. Archibald KC, Vignos Jr PJ. A study of contractures in muscular dystrophy. Arch Phys Med Rehabil. 1959;40(4):150–7.
37. Johnson EW, Kennedy JH. Comprehensive management of Duchenne muscular dystrophy. Arch Phys Med Rehabil. 1971;52(3):110–4.
38. Iannaccone ST, Russman BS, Browne RH, Buncher CR, White M, Samaha FJ. Prospective analysis of strength in spinal muscular atrophy. DCN/Spinal Muscular Atrophy Group. J Child Neurol. 2000;15(2):97–101.
39. Bodor M, McDonald CM. Why short stature is beneficial in Duchenne muscular dystrophy. Muscle Nerve. 2013;48(3):336–42.
40. Bushby K. Diagnosis and management of the limb girdle muscular dystrophies. Pract Neurol. 2009;9(6):314–23.
41. Janssen BH, Voet NB, Nabuurs CI, et al. Distinct disease phases in muscles of facioscapulohumeral dystrophy patients identified by MR detected fat infiltration. PLoS One. 2014;9(1):e85416.
42. Bergsma A, Murgia A, Cup EH, Verstegen PP, Meijer K, de Groot IJ. Upper extremity kinematics and muscle activation patterns in subjects with facioscapulohumeral dystrophy. Arch Phys Med Rehabil. 2014;95(9):1731–41.
43. Bergsma A, Cup EH, Geurts AC, de Groot IJ. Upper extremity function and activity in facioscapulohumeral dystrophy and limb-girdle muscular dystrophies: a systematic review. Disabil Rehabil. 2014;7:1–16.
44. Vignos Jr PJ, Spencer Jr GE, Archibald KC. Management of progressive muscular dystrophy in childhood. JAMA. 1963;184:89–96.
45. Vignos Jr PJ. Physical models of rehabilitation in neuromuscular disease. Muscle Nerve. 1983;6(5):323–38.
46. Johnson EW. Controversies about Duchenne muscular dystrophy. Dev Med Child Neurol. 1980;22(3):401–2.
47. King W, Pandya S. Physical therapy & FSHD—a guide for patients and physical therapists. Lexington: FSH Society; 2009.
48. Tawil R, McDermott MP, Mendell JR, Kissel J, Griggs RC. Facioscapulohumeral muscular dystrophy (FSHD): design of natural history study and results of baseline testing. FSH-DY Group. Neurology. 1994;44(3 Pt 1):442–6.
49. Kissel JT. Facioscapulohumeral dystrophy. Semin Neurol. 1999;19(1):35–43.
50. Statland JM, McDermott MP, Heatwole C, et al. Reevaluating measures of disease progression in facioscapulohumeral muscular dystrophy. Neuromuscul Disord. 2013;23(4):306–12.
51. Tawil R, van der Maarel SM, Tapscott SJ. Facioscapulohumeral dystrophy: the path to consensus on pathophysiology. Skelet Muscle. 2014;4:12.
52. Emery AE. Emery-Dreifuss muscular dystrophy and other related disorders. Br Med Bull. 1989;45(3):772–87.
53. Emery AE. Emery-Dreifuss muscular dystrophy—a 40 year retrospective. Neuromuscul Disord. 2000;10(4–5):228–32.
54. Merlini L. Selectivity of muscle sparing in Emery-Dreifuss muscular dystrophy. Neuromuscul Disord. 2009;19(7):500–1.
55. Vignos PJ, Wagner MB, Karlinchak B, Katirji B. Evaluation of a program for long-term treatment of Duchenne muscular dystrophy. Experience at the University Hospitals of Cleveland. J Bone Joint Surg Am. 1996;78(12):1844–52.
56. Kishnani PS, Steiner RD, Bali D, et al. Pompe disease diagnosis and management guideline. Genet Med. 2006;8(5):267–88.
57. Wang CH, Finkel RS, Bertini ES, et al. Consensus statement for standard of care in spinal muscular atrophy. J Child Neurol. 2007;22(8):1027–49.

58. World Health Organization. International classification of functioning, disability, and health (ICF). Geneva: World Health Organization; 2001.
59. Carter GT, Weiss MD, Chamberlain JR, et al. Aging with muscular dystrophy: pathophysiology and clinical management. Phys Med Rehabil Clin N Am. 2010;21(2):429–50.
60. Mercuri E, Mayhew A, Muntoni F, et al. Towards harmonisation of outcome measures for DMD and SMA within TREAT-NMD; report of three expert workshops: TREAT-NMD/ ENMC workshop on outcome measures, 12th–13th May 2007, Naarden, The Netherlands; TREAT-NMD workshop on outcome measures in experimental trials for DMD, 30th June– 1st July 2007, Naarden, The Netherlands; conjoint Institute of Myology TREAT-NMD meeting on physical activity monitoring in neuromuscular disorders, 11th July 2007, Paris, France. Neuromuscul Disord. 2008;18(11):894–903.
61. Brooke MH, Griggs RC, Mendell JR, Fenichel GM, Shumate JB, Pellegrino RJ. Clinical trial in Duchenne dystrophy. I. The design of the protocol. Muscle Nerve. 1981;4(3):186–97.
62. Haley SM, Coster WJ, Ludlow LH, et al. The pediatric evaluation of disability inventory. Boston: Center for Rehabilitation Effectiveness, Boston University; 1992.
63. Varni JW, Seid M, Rode CA. The PedsQL: measurement model for the pediatric quality of life inventory. Med Care. 1999;37(2):126–39.
64. Krupp LB, LaRocca NG, Muir-Nash J, Steinberg AD. The fatigue severity scale. Application to patients with multiple sclerosis and systemic lupus erythematosus. Arch Neurol. 1989;46(10):1121–3.
65. Brooke MH, Miller R. Fatigue testing. Muscle Nerve. 1990;13(Suppl):S35–7.
66. Learmonth YC, Dlugonski D, Pilutti LA, Sandroff BM, Klaren R, Motl RW. Psychometric properties of the Fatigue Severity Scale and the Modified Fatigue Impact Scale. J Neurol Sci. 2013;331(1–2):102–7.
67. McDonald CM, Henricson EK, Abresch RT, et al. The 6-minute walk test and other clinical endpoints in Duchenne muscular dystrophy: reliability, concurrent validity, and minimal clinically important differences from a multicenter study. Muscle Nerve. 2013;48(3): 357–68.
68. McDonald CM, Henricson EK, Abresch RT, et al. The 6-minute walk test and other endpoints in Duchenne muscular dystrophy: longitudinal natural history observations over 48 weeks from a multicenter study. Muscle Nerve. 2013;48(3):343–56.
69. Keith RA, Granger CV, Hamilton BB, Sherwin FS. The functional independence measure: a new tool for rehabilitation. Adv Clin Rehabil. 1987;1:6–18.
70. Ottenbacher KJ, Msall ME, Lyon NR, Duffy LC, Granger CV, Braun S. Interrater agreement and stability of the Functional Independence Measure for Children (WeeFIM): use in children with developmental disabilities. Arch Phys Med Rehabil. 1997;78(12):1309–15.
71. Lerman JA, Sullivan E, Haynes RJ. The Pediatric Outcomes Data Collection Instrument (PODCI) and functional assessment in patients with adolescent or juvenile idiopathic scoliosis and congenital scoliosis or kyphosis. Spine (Phila Pa 1976). 2002;27(18):2052–7. Discussion 2057–8.
72. Lerman JA, Sullivan E, Barnes DA, Haynes RJ. The Pediatric Outcomes Data Collection Instrument (PODCI) and functional assessment of patients with unilateral upper extremity deficiencies. J Pediatr Orthop. 2005;25(3):405–7.
73. Lee KM, Chung CY, Park MS, et al. Level of improvement determined by PODCI is related to parental satisfaction after single-event multilevel surgery in children with cerebral palsy. J Pediatr Orthop. 2010;30(4):396–402.
74. Klepper SE. Measures of pediatric function: Child Health Assessment Questionnaire (C-HAQ), Juvenile Arthritis Functional Assessment Scale (JAFAS), Pediatric Outcomes Data Collection Instrument (PODCI), and Activities Scale for Kids (ASK). Arthritis Care Res (Hoboken). 2011;63 Suppl 11:S371–82.
75. Gates PE, Otsuka NY, Sanders JO, McGee-Brown J. Relationship between parental PODCI questionnaire and School Function Assessment in measuring performance in children with CP. Dev Med Child Neurol. 2008;50(9):690–5.

76. Gates PE, Campbell SR. Effects of age, sex, and comorbidities on the Pediatric Outcomes Data Collection Instrument (PODCI) in the general population. J Pediatr Orthop. 2015;35(2): 203–9.

77. Ward DS, Bar-Or O. Use of the Borg scale in exercise prescription for overweight youth. Can J Sport Sci. 1990;15(2):120–5.

78. Wilson RC, Jones PW. Long-term reproducibility of Borg scale estimates of breathlessness during exercise. Clin Sci (Lond). 1991;80(4):309–12.

79. Hommerding PX, Donadio MV, Paim TF, Marostica PJ. The Borg scale is accurate in children and adolescents older than 9 years with cystic fibrosis. Respir Care. 2010;55(6):729–33.

80. Florence JM, Pandya S, King WM, et al. Intrarater reliability of manual muscle test (Medical Research Council scale) grades in Duchenne's muscular dystrophy. Phys Ther. 1992;72(2):115–22. Discussion 122–116.

81. Escolar DM, Henricson EK, Mayhew J, et al. Clinical evaluator reliability for quantitative and manual muscle testing measures of strength in children. Muscle Nerve. 2001;24(6): 787–93.

82. Angelini C, Semplicini C, Tonin P, et al. Progress in enzyme replacement therapy in glycogen storage disease type II. Ther Adv Neurol Disord. 2009;2(3):143–53.

83. Angelini C, Semplicini C, Ravaglia S, et al. New motor outcome function measures in evaluation of late-onset Pompe disease before and after enzyme replacement therapy. Muscle Nerve. 2012;45(6):831–4.

84. Hagemans ML, Laforet P, Hop WJ, et al. Impact of late-onset Pompe disease on participation in daily life activities: evaluation of the Rotterdam Handicap Scale. Neuromuscul Disord. 2007;17(7):537–43.

85. McColl MA, Paterson M, Davies D, Doubt L, Law M. Validity and community utility of the Canadian Occupational Performance Measure. Can J Occup Ther. 2000;67(1):22–30.

86. Law M, Baptiste S, McColl M, Opzoomer A, Polatajko H, Pollock N. The Canadian occupational performance measure: an outcome measure for occupational therapy. Can J Occup Ther. 1990;57(2):82–7.

87. Wilson RC, Jones PW. A comparison of the visual analogue scale and modified Borg scale for the measurement of dyspnoea during exercise. Clin Sci (Lond). 1989;76(3):277–82.

88. Mazzone ES, Messina S, Vasco G, et al. Reliability of the North Star Ambulatory Assessment in a multicentric setting. Neuromuscul Disord. 2009;19(7):458–61.

89. Mazzone E, Martinelli D, Berardinelli A, et al. North Star Ambulatory Assessment, 6-minute walk test and timed items in ambulant boys with Duchenne muscular dystrophy. Neuromuscul Disord. 2010;20(11):712–6.

90. Mayhew A, Cano S, Scott E, Eagle M, Bushby K, Muntoni F. Moving towards meaningful measurement: Rasch analysis of the North Star Ambulatory Assessment in Duchenne muscular dystrophy. Dev Med Child Neurol. 2011;53(6):535–42.

91. Ergul Y, Ekici B, Nisli K, et al. Evaluation of the North Star Ambulatory Assessment scale and cardiac abnormalities in ambulant boys with Duchenne muscular dystrophy. J Paediatr Child Health. 2012;48(7):610–6.

92. Mayhew AG, Cano SJ, Scott E, et al. Detecting meaningful change using the North Star Ambulatory Assessment in Duchenne muscular dystrophy. Dev Med Child Neurol. 2013; 55(11):1046–52.

93. De Sanctis R, Pane M, Sivo S, et al. Suitability of North Star Ambulatory Assessment in young boys with Duchenne muscular dystrophy. Neuromuscul Disord. 2015;25(1):14–8.

94. Raat H, Bonsel GJ, Essink-Bot ML, Landgraf JM, Gemke RJ. Reliability and validity of comprehensive health status measures in children: The Child Health Questionnaire in relation to the Health Utilities Index. J Clin Epidemiol. 2002;55(1):67–76.

95. Berard C, Payan C, Hodgkinson I, Fermanian J. A motor function measure for neuromuscular diseases. Construction and validation study. Neuromuscul Disord. 2005;15(7):463–70.

96. Young NL, Williams JI, Yoshida KK, Wright JG. Measurement properties of the activities scale for kids. J Clin Epidemiol. 2000;53(2):125–37.

97. Young NL, Varni JW, Snider L, et al. The Internet is valid and reliable for child-report: an example using the Activities Scale for Kids (ASK) and the Pediatric Quality of Life Inventory (PedsQL). J Clin Epidemiol. 2009;62(3):314–20.

98. Main M, Kairon H, Mercuri E, Muntoni F. The Hammersmith functional motor scale for children with spinal muscular atrophy: a scale to test ability and monitor progress in children with limited ambulation. Eur J Paediatr Neurol. 2003;7(4):155–9.

99. Krosschell KJ, Maczulski JA, Crawford TO, Scott C, Swoboda KJ. A modified Hammersmith functional motor scale for use in multi-center research on spinal muscular atrophy. Neuromuscul Disord. 2006;16(7):417–26.

100. van Capelle CI, van der Beek NA, de Vries JM, et al. The quick motor function test: a new tool to rate clinical severity and motor function in Pompe patients. J Inherit Metab Dis. 2012;35(2):317–23.

101. McDonald CM, Widman LM, Walsh DD, Walsh SA, Abresch RT. Use of step activity monitoring for continuous physical activity assessment in boys with Duchenne muscular dystrophy. Arch Phys Med Rehabil. 2005;86(4):802–8.

102. McDonald CM, Widman L, Abresch RT, Walsh SA, Walsh DD. Utility of a step activity monitor for the measurement of daily ambulatory activity in children. Arch Phys Med Rehabil. 2005;86(4):793–801.

103. Steffensen B, Hyde S, Lyager S, Mattsson E. Validity of the EK scale: a functional assessment of non-ambulatory individuals with Duchenne muscular dystrophy or spinal muscular atrophy. Physiother Res Int. 2001;6(3):119–34.

104. Piper MC, Darrah J. Motor assessment of the developing infant. Philadelphia: W. B. Saunders; 1994.

105. Russell D, Rosenbaum P, Avery L, Lane M. Gross motor function measure (GMFM-66 & GMFM-88) user's manual. London: Mac Keith; 2002.

106. Folio MR, Fewell R. Peabody developmental motor scales. 2nd ed. Austin: Pro-Ed; 2000.

107. Bruininks R. Bruininks-Oseretsky test of motor proficiency. 2nd ed. Minneapolis: Pearson; 2005.

108. Mayhew A, Mazzone ES, Eagle M, et al. Development of the performance of the upper limb module for Duchenne muscular dystrophy. Dev Med Child Neurol. 2013;55(11):1038–45.

109. ATS Committee on Proficiency Standards for Clinical Pulmonary Function Laboratories. ATS statement: guidelines for the six-minute walk test. Am J Respir Crit Care Med. 2002;166(1):111–7.

110. Fairbank JC, Couper J, Davies JB, O'Brien JP. The Oswestry low back pain disability questionnaire. Physiotherapy. 1980;66(8):271–3.

111. Bieri D, Reeve RA, Champion GD, Addicoat L, Ziegler JB. The Faces Pain Scale for the self-assessment of the severity of pain experienced by children: development, initial validation, and preliminary investigation for ratio scale properties. Pain. 1990;41(2):139–50.

112. Krechel SW, Bildner J. CRIES: a new neonatal postoperative pain measurement score. Initial testing of validity and reliability. Paediatr Anaesth. 1995;5(1):53–61.

113. Pasero CL. Using the Faces scale to assess pain. Am J Nurs. 1997;97(7):19–20.

114. Ferrell BA, Stein WM, Beck JC. The Geriatric Pain Measure: validity, reliability and factor analysis. J Am Geriatr Soc. 2000;48(12):1669–73.

115. McCaffery M. Choosing a faces pain scale. Nursing. 2002;32(5):68.

116. O'Rourke D. The measurement of pain in infants, children, and adolescents: from policy to practice. Phys Ther. 2004;84(6):560–70.

117. Salaffi F, Stancati A, Silvestri CA, Ciapetti A, Grassi W. Minimal clinically important changes in chronic musculoskeletal pain intensity measured on a numerical rating scale. Eur J Pain. 2004;8(4):283–91.

118. Tashjian RZ, Deloach J, Porucznik CA, Powell AP. Minimal clinically important differences (MCID) and patient acceptable symptomatic state (PASS) for visual analog scales (VAS) measuring pain in patients treated for rotator cuff disease. J Shoulder Elbow Surg. 2009;18(6):927–32.

119. McDonald CM. Limb contractures in progressive neuromuscular disease and the role of stretching, orthotics, and surgery. Phys Med Rehabil Clin N Am. 1998;9(1):187–211.
120. Siegel IM. Plastic-molded knee-ankle-foot orthoses in the treatment of Duchenne muscular dystrophy. Arch Phys Med Rehabil. 1975;56(7):322.
121. Siegel IM. Prolongation of ambulation through early percutaneous tenotomy and bracing with plastic orthoses. Isr J Med Sci. 1977;13(2):192–6.
122. Aprile I, Bordieri C, Gilardi A, et al. Balance and walking involvement in facioscapulo-humeral dystrophy: a pilot study on the effects of custom lower limb orthoses. Eur J Phys Rehabil Med. 2013;49(2):169–78.
123. Hyde SA, FlLytrup I, Glent S, et al. A randomized comparative study of two methods for controlling Tendo Achilles contracture in Duchenne muscular dystrophy. Neuromuscul Disord. 2000;10(4–5):257–63.
124. Ward K, Alsop C, Caulton J, Rubin C, Adams J, Mughal Z. Low magnitude mechanical loading is osteogenic in children with disabling conditions. J Bone Miner Res. 2004;19(3):360–9.
125. Ashmore CR, Lee YB, Summers P, Hitchcock L. Stretch-induced growth in chicken wing muscles: nerve-muscle interaction in muscular dystrophy. Am J Physiol. 1984;246(5 Pt 1):C378–84.
126. Glanzman AM, Flickinger JM, Dholakia KH, Bonnemann CG, Finkel RS. Serial casting for the management of ankle contracture in Duchenne muscular dystrophy. Pediatr Phys Ther. 2011;23(3):275–9.
127. Main M, Mercuri E, Haliloglu G, Baker R, Kinali M, Muntoni F. Serial casting of the ankles in Duchenne muscular dystrophy: can it be an alternative to surgery? Neuromuscul Disord. 2007;17(3):227–30.
128. American Physical Therapy Association. Guide to physical therapy practice. Phys Ther. 2001;81(1).
129. Townsend EL, Tamhane H, Gross KD. Effects of AFO use on walking in boys with Duchenne muscular dystrophy: a pilot study. Pediatr Phys Ther. 2015;27(1):24–9.
130. Chyatte SB, Long II C, Vignos Jr PJ. The balanced forearm orthosis in muscular dystrophy. Arch Phys Med Rehabil. 1965;46(9):633–6.
131. Han JJ, Kurillo G, Abresch RT, de Bie E, Nicorici A, Bajcsy R. Reachable workspace in facioscapulohumeral muscular dystrophy (FSHD) by Kinect. Muscle Nerve. 2015;51(2):168–75.
132. Han JJ, Kurillo G, Abresch RT, Nicorici A, Bajcsy R. Validity, reliability, and sensitivity of a 3D vision sensor-based upper extremity reachable workspace evaluation in neuromuscular diseases. PLoS Curr. 2013;5.
133. Vignos Jr PJ, Archibald KC. Maintenance of ambulation in childhood muscular dystrophy. J Chronic Dis. 1960;12:273–90.
134. Spencer Jr GE, Vignos Jr PJ. Bracing for ambulation in childhood progressive muscular dystrophy. Am J Orthop. 1962;44-A:234–42.
135. Vignos Jr PJ, Wagner MB, Kaplan JS, Spencer Jr GE. Predicting the success of reambulation in patients with Duchenne muscular dystrophy. J Bone Joint Surg Am. 1983;65(6):719–28.
136. Bowker JH, Halpin PJ. Factors determining success in reambulation of the child with progressive muscular dystrophy. Orthop Clin North Am. 1978;9(2):431–6.
137. Tardieu C, Lespargot A, Tabary C, Bret MD. For how long must the soleus muscle be stretched each day to prevent contracture? Dev Med Child Neurol. 1988;30(1):3–10.
138. Stuberg WA. Considerations related to weight-bearing programs in children with developmental disabilities. Phys Ther. 1992;72(1):35–40.
139. Spencer Jr GE. Orthopaedic care of progressive muscular dystrophy. J Bone Joint Surg Am. 1967;49(6):1201–4.
140. Alman BA, Raza SN, Biggar WD. Steroid treatment and the development of scoliosis in males with Duchenne muscular dystrophy. J Bone Joint Surg Am. 2004;86-A(3):519–24.
141. Brooke MH, Fenichel GM, Griggs RC, et al. Duchenne muscular dystrophy: patterns of clinical progression and effects of supportive therapy. Neurology. 1989;39(4):475–81.

142. Smith AD, Koreska J, Moseley CF. Progression of scoliosis in Duchenne muscular dystrophy. J Bone Joint Surg Am. 1989;71(7):1066–74.
143. Siegel IM. Spinal stabilization in Duchenne muscular dystrophy: rationale and method. Muscle Nerve. 1982;5(5):417–8.
144. Gardner-Medwin D. Controversies about Duchenne muscular dystrophy. (2) Bracing for ambulation. Dev Med Child Neurol. 1979;21(5):659–62.
145. Kerr TP, Lin JP, Gresty MA, Morley T, Robb SA. Spinal stability is improved by inducing a lumbar lordosis in boys with Duchenne muscular dystrophy: a pilot study. Gait Posture. 2008;28(1):108–12.
146. Kinali M, Main M, Eliahoo J, et al. Predictive factors for the development of scoliosis in Duchenne muscular dystrophy. Eur J Paediatr Neurol. 2007;11(3):160–6.
147. Muntoni F, Bushby K, Manzur AY. Muscular dystrophy campaign funded workshop on management of scoliosis in Duchenne muscular dystrophy 24 January 2005, London, UK. Neuromuscul Disord. 2006;16(3):210–9.
148. Rodillo EB, Fernandez-Bermejo E, Heckmatt JZ, Dubowitz V. Prevention of rapidly progressive scoliosis in Duchenne muscular dystrophy by prolongation of walking with orthoses. J Child Neurol. 1988;3(4):269–74.
149. Siegel IM. The management of muscular dystrophy: a clinical review. Muscle Nerve. 1978;1(6):453–60.
150. Wilkins KE, Gibson DA. The patterns of spinal deformity in Duchenne muscular dystrophy. J Bone Joint Surg Am. 1976;58(1):24–32.
151. Case LE. Physical therapy management of the spine in Duchenne muscular dystrophy. Postgraduate fellowship project, Postgraduate fellowship in pediatric physical and occupational therapy, University of North Carolina at Chapel Hill. 1985.
152. Johnson EW, Yarnell SK. Hand dominance and scoliosis in Duchenne muscular dystrophy. Arch Phys Med Rehabil. 1976;57(10):462–4.
153. Johnson EW, Walter J. Zeiter Lecture: pathokinesiology of Duchenne muscular dystrophy: implications for management. Arch Phys Med Rehabil. 1977;58(1):4–7.
154. Gibson DA, Albisser AM, Koreska J. Role of the wheelchair in the management of the muscular dystrophy patient. Can Med Assoc J. 1975;113(10):964–6.
155. Gibson DA, Wilkins KE. The management of spinal deformities in Duchenne muscular dystrophy. A new concept of spinal bracing. Clin Orthop Relat Res. 1975;108:41–51.
156. Koreska J, Robertson D, Mills RH, Gibson DA, Albisser AM. Biomechanics of the lumbar spine and its clinical significance. Orthop Clin North Am. 1977;8(1):121–33.
157. Werner BC, Skalsky AJ, McDonald CM, Han JJ. Convexity of scoliosis related to handedness in identical twin boys with Duchenne's muscular dystrophy: a case report. Arch Phys Med Rehabil. 2008;89(10):2021–4.
158. Bonsett CA. Prophylactic bracing in pseudohypertrophic muscular dystrophy (preliminary report) part I: patient experience. J Indiana State Med Assoc. 1975;68(3):181–4.
159. Bonsett CA, Glancy JJ. Prophylactic bracing in pseudohypertrophic muscular dystrophy (preliminary report). Part II: the brace. J Indiana State Med Assoc. 1975;68(3):185–7.
160. Brown JC, Zeller JL, Swank SM, Furumasu J, Warath SL. Surgical and functional results of spine fusion in spinal muscular atrophy. Spine. 1989;14(7):763–70.
161. Bleck EE. Mobility of patients with Duchenne muscular dystrophy. Dev Med Child Neurol. 1979;21(6):823–4.
162. Birnkrant DJ, Bushby KM, Amin RS, et al. The respiratory management of patients with Duchenne muscular dystrophy: a DMD care considerations working group specialty article. Pediatr Pulmonol. 2010;45(8):739–48.
163. Finder JD, Birnkrant D, Carl J, et al. Respiratory care of the patient with Duchenne muscular dystrophy: ATS consensus statement. Am J Respir Crit Care Med. 2004;170(4):456–65.
164. Eagle M, Baudouin SV, Chandler C, Giddings DR, Bullock R, Bushby K. Survival in Duchenne muscular dystrophy: improvements in life expectancy since 1967 and the impact of home nocturnal ventilation. Neuromuscul Disord. 2002;12(10):926–9.

165. ATS/ERS statement on respiratory muscle testing. Am J Respir Crit Care Med. 2002;166(4): 518–624.
166. Fauroux B, Quijano-Roy S, Desguerre I, Khirani S. The value of respiratory muscle testing in children with neuromuscular disease. Chest. 2015;147(2):552–9.
167. Topin N, Matecki S, Le Bris S, et al. Dose-dependent effect of individualized respiratory muscle training in children with Duchenne muscular dystrophy. Neuromuscul Disord. 2002;12(6):576–83.
168. Bushby K, Muntoni F, Bourke JP. 107th ENMC international workshop: the management of cardiac involvement in muscular dystrophy and myotonic dystrophy. 7th–9th June 2002, Naarden, The Netherlands. Neuromuscul Disord. 2003;13(2):166–72.
169. Takano N, Honke K, Hasui M, Ohno I, Takemura H. A case of pacemaker implantation for complete atrioventricular block associated with Duchenne muscular dystrophy. No To Hattatsu. 1997;29(6):476–80.
170. Cripe LH, Tobias JD. Cardiac considerations in the operative management of the patient with Duchenne or Becker muscular dystrophy. Paediatr Anaesth. 2013;23(9):777–84.
171. Yilmaz A, Sechtem U. Cardiac involvement in muscular dystrophy: advances in diagnosis and therapy. Heart. 2012;98(5):420–9.
172. Vignos Jr PJ, Watkins MP. The effect of exercise in muscular dystrophy. JAMA. 1966; 197(11):843–8.
173. Houser CR, Johnson DM. Breathing exercises for children with pseudohypertrophic muscular dystrophy. Phys Ther. 1971;51(7):751–9.
174. Fowler Jr WM, Taylor M. Rehabilitation management of muscular dystrophy and related disorders: I. The role of exercise. Arch Phys Med Rehabil. 1982;63(7):319–21.
175. Valentine BA, Blue JT, Cooper BJ. The effect of exercise on canine dystrophic muscle. Ann Neurol. 1989;26(4):588.
176. Armstrong RB, Warren GL, Warren JA. Mechanisms of exercise-induced muscle fibre injury. Sports Med. 1991;12(3):184–207.
177. McNeil PL, Khakee R. Disruptions of muscle fiber plasma membranes. Role in exercise-induced damage. Am J Pathol. 1992;140(5):1097–109.
178. Hayes A, Lynch GS, Williams DA. The effects of endurance exercise on dystrophic mdx mice. I. Contractile and histochemical properties of intact muscles. Proc R Soc Lond B Biol Sci. 1993;253(1336):19–25.
179. Lynch GS, Hayes A, Lam MH, Williams DA. The effects of endurance exercise on dystrophic mdx mice. II. Contractile properties of skinned muscle fibres. Proc Biol Sci. 1993;253(1336): 27–33.
180. Brussee V, Tardif F, Tremblay JP. Muscle fibers of mdx mice are more vulnerable to exercise than those of normal mice. Neuromuscul Disord. 1997;7(8):487–92.
181. Hayes A, Williams DA. Contractile function and low-intensity exercise effects of old dystrophic (mdx) mice. Am J Physiol. 1998;274(4 Pt 1):C1138–44.
182. Eagle M. Report on the muscular dystrophy campaign workshop: exercise in neuromuscular diseases Newcastle, January 2002. Neuromuscul Disord. 2002;12(10):975–83.
183. Fowler Jr WM. Role of physical activity and exercise training in neuromuscular diseases. Am J Phys Med Rehabil. 2002;81(11 Suppl):S187–95.
184. Abresch RT, Carter GT, Han JJ, McDonald CM. Exercise in neuromuscular diseases. Phys Med Rehabil Clin N Am. 2012;23(3):653–73.
185. Markert CD, Case LE, Carter GT, Furlong PA, Grange RW. Exercise and Duchenne muscular dystrophy: where we have been and where we need to go. Muscle Nerve. 2012;45(5):746–51.
186. Voet NB, Bleijenberg G, Padberg GW, van Engelen BG, Geurts AC. Effect of aerobic exercise training and cognitive behavioural therapy on reduction of chronic fatigue in patients with facioscapulohumeral dystrophy: protocol of the FACTS-2-FSHD trial. BMC Neurol. 2010;10:56.
187. Abresch RT, Han JJ, Carter GT. Rehabilitation management of neuromuscular disease: the role of exercise training. J Clin Neuromuscul Dis. 2009;11(1):7–21.

188. Rodillo E, Noble-Jamieson CM, Aber V, Heckmatt JZ, Muntoni F, Dubowitz V. Respiratory muscle training in Duchenne muscular dystrophy. Arch Dis Child. 1989;64(5):736–8.

189. Gozal D, Thiriet P. Respiratory muscle training in neuromuscular disease: long-term effects on strength and load perception. Med Sci Sports Exerc. 1999;31(11):1522–7.

190. Estrup C, Lyager S, Noeraa N, Olsen C. Effect of respiratory muscle training in patients with neuromuscular diseases and in normals. Respiration. 1986;50(1):36–43.

191. Smith PE, Coakley JH, Edwards RH. Respiratory muscle training in Duchenne muscular dystrophy. Muscle Nerve. 1988;11(7):784–5.

192. Aslan GK, Gurses HN, Issever H, Kiyan E. Effects of respiratory muscle training on pulmonary functions in patients with slowly progressive neuromuscular disease: a randomized controlled trial. Clin Rehabil. 2013;28(6):573–81.

193. Peltekova I, Storr M. Case 1: back pain in a boy with Duchenne muscular dystrophy. Paediatr Child Health. 2014;19(6):299–300.

# Chapter 9
# Orthopaedic Management of the Child with Muscular Dystrophy

**Robert K. Lark and Elizabeth W. Hubbard**

## Introduction

The orthopaedic care of children with muscular dystrophy (MD) is a challenging endeavor. Although many similarities exist, each subtype of MD can present differently. It is imperative that the proper diagnosis be confirmed so that treatment can be initiated based on knowledge of the natural history of the disease. Advancements in the medical management of MD are challenging historic recommendations for orthopaedic care. This chapter is intended to provide a brief, general overview of orthopaedic management of the most common childhood MDs.

## Duchenne Muscular Dystrophy

Duchenne muscular dystrophy (DMD) is the most common childhood MD. As diagnostic genetic testing continues to improve, referral to the orthopaedic surgeon for consideration of muscle biopsy may be on the decline. Orthopaedic manifestations of this disease include gait abnormality, muscle weakness/imbalance, joint contractures, fractures, and scoliosis.

R.K. Lark, M.D., M.S. • E. Hubbard, M.D. (✉)
Department of Orthopaedic Surgery, Duke University Medical Center,
Lenox Baker Children's Hospital, 3000 Erwin Rd,
Durham, NC 27705, USA
e-mail: elizabeth.hubbard@duke.edu

© Springer International Publishing Switzerland 2015
R.A. Huml (ed.), *Muscular Dystrophy*, DOI 10.1007/978-3-319-17362-7_9

## Non-operative Management

Although not necessarily applicable to other forms of MD, steroids (i.e. deflazacort, prednisone) are showing promise for prolonging ambulatory ability and decreasing the rate of scoliosis [1–4]. Unfortunately, side effects such as obesity, osteopenia, and fractures may negate some of the positive attributes of the drugs [5–7]. Studies are ongoing to determine the appropriate dosing regimen and duration of steroid treatment as cessation of the drug seems to lead to rapid decline of muscle strength [1, 3].

A common presentation to the orthopaedic surgeon is for evaluation of toe walking in early childhood, often in the three- to five-year age range. Careful assessment of the child's birth history and complete musculoskeletal physical exam is essential to rule out other causes such as idiopathic toe walking, cerebral palsy, etc. It is not uncommon for these children to have a mild equinus contracture at this age and physical therapy can aid in maintaining ankle joint range of motion. Serial casting may also be considered followed by maintenance of foot position with an ankle foot orthosis [8]. As the child continues to grow, hamstring and hip flexion contractures worsen as the proximal muscles weaken. Continued stretching and consideration of a knee-ankle-foot orthosis may be considered to prolong ambulation and standing ability [9–11]. Contractures also occur in the upper extremities and may require occupational therapy evaluation for stretching and assistive devices to aid in activities of daily living [12–14].

Patients not receiving steroids have a high incidence of developing scoliosis. Once confined to a wheelchair, thoracic supports may aid in maintaining sitting posture, but likely do not impact progression of the curve. Bracing is not indicated as the efficacy of brace treatment has not been shown to be beneficial in this condition [15–20].

Fractures are common once ambulatory ability is lost [5–7, 21]. Most fractures occur about the knee (most commonly the distal femur). Fracture management typically is non-operative. Care should be taken to avoid rigid immobilization with a heavy fiberglass or plaster cast as this can cause a fracture at the proximal end of the wrap. Most children are comfortable in a bulky wrap for four to six weeks until signs of radiographic union are evident. Bisphosphonates have been shown to improve back pain in patients with vertebral fractures, but have not been shown to decrease fracture risk [6].

## Operative Management

When conservative measures fail, operative management of children with DMD can be beneficial. Clear goals of the surgical procedure must be discussed with and understood by the family. Shapiro et al. proposed a system of surgical approaches based on the ambulatory ability of the patient [9]. The three basic categories include ambulatory, rehabilitative, and palliative. The ambulatory category was subdivided into early-extensive, moderate, and minimum ambulatory approaches. The early-extensive approach is intended to be performed while the patient remains ambulatory and attempts to prevent the extensive contractures around the hip, knee, and ankle. The procedure involves excising the tensor fascia, lengthening the hip flexors, hamstrings, Achilles tendon, and possibly transferring the posterior tibialis through the inter-osseus membrane to the dorsum of the foot. While early reports of this method were promising, longer follow-up studies have failed to show much benefit. The "moderate ambulatory approach" is intended to address existing contractures in hopes to maintain ambulatory ability. The approach is similar to the extensive approach by utilizing intramuscular lengthening techniques of the gastrosoleus complex as well as lengthening the hamstrings. The lengthening of hip flexors and tensor fasciae showed no increased benefit. The minimum ambulatory approach addresses only the equinus contracture. An intramuscular approach such as the Vulpius lengthening is recommended to minimize the risk of over-lengthening potential that can occur with a z-lengthening. The rehabilitative approach is intended to allow a child with recent loss of ambulation to regain the ability to walk. This involves addressing the hip and knee contractures as well as percutaneously tenotomizing the Achilles. This approach requires post-operative brace management, but has been reported to increase ambulatory ability from several months to a few years. The palliative approach addresses the severe equinus deformity that prevents the patient from achieving a plantigrade foot to rest on the plate of his wheelchair. The procedure involves tenotomies of the Achilles, flexor digitorum, and flexor hallucis longus as well as tenotomy vs. transfer of the posterior tibialis to the dorsum of the foot [22, 23].

In the event the patient develops scoliosis, it should be addressed quickly (Cobb angle >20°) as it remains unclear which patients will progress [20, 24]. Bracing is ineffective in this condition. Delaying surgery may unintentionally cause the child to have to forego spinal fusion due to decline in pulmonary reserve [20, 24]. Surgical correction of scoliosis in patients with DMD has generated much debate. Instrumentation must be individualized to each patient and may include pedicle screw fixation, sublaminar wires, hooks, or a combination of anchors. Patients with pelvic obliquity should be fused to the pelvis, whereas those with a level pelvis may have success stopping at L5 [25–27]. The patient and family should be warned of potential risks such as bleeding, prolonged intubation, and infection. Additionally, children with moderate to severe upper extremity weakness may no longer be able to feed themselves as they lose the ability to move their trunk to their hands [28, 29].

## Becker Muscular Dystrophy

Becker muscular dystrophy (BMD) is a less severe dystrophinopathy compared to Duchenne. These children ambulate for a longer duration and may never become confined to a wheelchair. Scoliosis is infrequent in this population.

## *Non-operative Management*

As with Duchenne, corticosteroids play a role in the non-operative treatment of BMD. Johnsen [30] reported that two patients with Becker's had a significant improvement in overall strength and reduction in serum creatine kinase levels after therapeutic treatment with prednisone. Because the severity of the disease varies with the level of functional dystrophin protein that is expressed, patients with BMD can differ in the clinical manifestations of the disease. Further studies are required in this patient population to determine which subset of patient's with BMD would best benefit from prolonged corticosteroid treatment.

Patients with BMD often remain ambulatory longer and have an overall slower disease course than patients with DMD. Orthoses can be beneficial in patients who develop ankle and forefoot equinus [31]. Patients with BMD are felt to be better candidates for bracing than patients with Duchenne, both because they remain ambulatory and retain muscle strength longer.

## *Operative Management*

Patients with BMD can develop similar orthopaedic conditions as those with Duchenne. However, the manifestations are typically delayed and less severe. The need for and timing of surgical intervention for orthopaedic manifestations of Becker's is both reduced and delayed when compared with patients who have DMD [32].

Forefoot and ankle equinus have been described in these patients. When refractory to stretching and orthoses, intramuscular lengthening of the Achilles tendon is effective for management of ankle equinus [33]. Patients should also undergo concurrent posterior tibialis tendon transfer to the dorsum of the foot if appropriate [32, 33].

Scoliosis is seen more commonly in non-ambulatory adolescents. Because most patients with BMD remain ambulatory through adolescence and into adulthood, fewer patients develop scoliosis in adolescence [32]. Patients with BMD are still at greater risk for scolisosis overall and should be monitored closely with serial exams. As with patients who have DMD, patients with BMD should be considered surgical candidates when curves progress beyond 20° and the surgical principles are the same for both conditions [34].

## Facioscapulohumeral Muscular Dystrophy

Facioscapulohumeral muscular dystrophy (FSHD) is an autosomal dominant disorder resulting in progressive weakness of the shoulder girdle and facial musculature. Orthopaedic manifestations include severe shoulder weakness, hyperlordosis, and eventually gait abnormalities. Scoliosis is rare but does occur.

## Non-operative Management

Non-operative approaches to the management of FSHD have evolved over recent years. Early literature reported that muscle strengthening placed patients at risk for disease progression due to destruction of muscle fibers. However, more recent literature has shown that strength training and physical therapy can have positive effects. Andersen et al. showed that creatine kinase levels normalize within 24 h compared with pre-exercise levels, suggesting that irreversible or prolonged muscle damage is not an effect of exercise in these patients [35]. Olsen et al. found that a three-month low-intensity aerobic training program both improved oxygen uptake and caused no evidence of muscle damage among patients with FSHD [36]. Bakhtiary et al. attempted to optimize muscle function and found that simple motor learning programs could help FSHD patients adopt more effective muscle performance during basic tasks that require shoulder abduction and elbow flexion [37].

Taking things a step further, Pasotti et al. designed a six-month exercise and nutrition supplement program for a 43-year-old patient with FSHD [38]. At the time of the initiation of the program, the patient was noted to have severe proximal muscle weakness, hyperlordosis, and was no longer ambulatory. Pulmonary function tests revealed mild restrictive lung disease. The patient began a regimen of both endurance and strength training. Her diet was supplemented with branched chain amino acids, creatinine, and conjugated linoleic acid, based on previously published data that these agents can limit exercise-induced injury [39–41]. The patient developed a modest increase in shoulder abduction strength, with improvement in body mass composition and stabilization of pulmonary function tests, with no evidence of muscle soreness or muscle destruction [38].

There is also growing literature on the effects of albuterol as a potential adjunct in the treatment regimen for patients with facioscapulohumeral dystrophy. A pilot trial of 15 patients with FSHD shows that daily treatments of sustained-release albuterol over a three-month period significantly improved patients' lean body mass and strength [42]. A follow-up randomized clinical trial involving 90 FSHD patients showed that daily treatment with long-acting albuterol resulted in improved grip strength and significantly improved muscle mass, although global measures of muscle strength did not significantly improve [43]. Albuterol was relatively well-tolerated by the patients in the study and the authors suggested that combining albuterol with other treatment modalities, such as strength training programs, might result in more significant anabolic effects.

## Operative Management

Surgical management of facioscapulohumeral dystrophy is largely directed at scapular stabilization. The manifestation of FSHD that mostly limits daily activities is the patient's inability to abduct his or her shoulders. Weakness of the trapezius, rhomboids, levator scapulae, and subscapularis causes significant scapular winging with any attempt at shoulder abduction. Stabilizing the scapula against the thoracic wall allows the deltoid and supraspinatus to abduct and forward flex the upper extremity. The shoulder range of motion achieved with stabilization is still less compared to that of unaffected patients, but the motion and strength is significantly improved post-operatively for patients with FSHD. Stabilization can be done either through scapulopexy or scapulothoracic arthrodesis.

Scapulopexy involves stabilizing the scapula against the thoracic cavity without attempting to achieve an arthrodesis. This can be achieved by using autograft, such as fascia lata graft, or other materials such as merseline tape, dacron, or looped wire [44, 45]. The procedure requires minimal post-operative immobilization. After surgery, patients can begin immediate shoulder range of motion. Because immediate range of motion is encouraged, patients can undergo contemporaneous bilateral scapulopexy or briefly stage the procedure so that both shoulders can be addressed. Ketenjian suggested that scapulopexy should be the preferred treatment in patients with FSHD because it does not interfere with rib excursion and therefore would not have significant negative effects on pulmonary function [45]. He reported improved shoulder abduction of an average 33°, as well as improvement in strength, endurance, pain, and cosmesis in five patients who underwent scapulopexy. Average patient follow-up in this study was 34 months. Giannini et al. reported significant improvements in both shoulder abduction and forward flexion in 10 patients who underwent scapulopexy for FSHD. The scapulae were fixed to the underlying fourth through seventh ribs using wires passed through bone tunnels. Although initial results were good, average forward flexion and muscle strength declined during long-term follow-up [44].

Scapulothoracic arthrodesis is a more technically demanding procedure than scapulopexy. The goal is to fuse the scapula to the underlying ribs. Numerous techniques have been described, although many follow a similar surgical plan [46–55]. Authors recommend making a posterior incision and elevating the rhomboids and trapezius off the medial border of the scapula, followed by a subperiosteal exposure of the underlying ribs [46, 48, 50, 55]. While most techniques recommend using iliac crest autograft, there are reports of successful arthrodesis using allograft [51]. Wires or multifilament cables are then threaded around the underlying ribs and attached to the scapula through bone tunnels, with more recently reported techniques recommending using a reconstruction or LCP plate to supplement scapular fixation and prevent scapular fracture and wire cut-out [47, 49, 54]. Most methods involve a post-operative immobilization period of 6–12 weeks to allow time for a successful fusion, although some authors encourage immediate range of motion post-operatively [50, 55]. Once shoulder range of motion is initiated, the rehabilitation protocol typically involves gentle range of motion passively, then actively, and then range of motion with weight bearing. The recovery time from this procedure is approximately six months. Simultaneous bilateral scapulothoracic arthrodesis is not encouraged because of the prolonged immobilization and weight-bearing restrictions post-operatively.

Both scapulopexy and scapulothoracic arthrodesis are complex procedures and a full pre-operative evaluation of the patient must be performed. Pre-operatively, the patient's passive and active shoulder abduction and forward flexion should be evaluated and recorded. The patient's active shoulder abduction and forward flexion should then be re-evaluated with the examiner stabilizing the patient's scapula. This is known as the Horwitz maneuver. With the examiner holding the patient's scapula, the deltoid and supraspinatus can contract against a stable scapula, allowing the muscles to abduct and forward flex the shoulder [33, 56]. Patients who will most benefit from a scapulopexy or scapulothoracic arthrodesis have active abduction and forward flexion from 90° to 120° when their scapulae are stabilized during the Horwitz maneuver. This represents the range of abduction required to carry out most activities of daily living [45]. Repeating the Horwitz maneuver with the scapula fixed at varying degrees of rotation against the thoracic wall can help determine the ideal position for scapular fixation intra-operatively by allowing the surgeon to see which scapula position gives the patient the optimal amount of shoulder motion.

When deciding between scapulopexy and scapulothoracic arthrodesis, the patient's pulmonary function and rate of disease progression should both be considered. Scapulopexy is a less invasive procedure and has been shown to have a less significant effect on a patient's pulmonary function, specifically forced vital capacity and overall vital capacity. This is even more important if the patient is considering bilateral procedures, as bilateral scapulothoracic arthrodesis has been shown to significantly affect pulmonary function both in the early recovery period and over the long-term follow-up. Also, patients with a rapidly progressive disease are likely better candidates for scapulopexy, as they would require less immobilization and would gain immediate function after the procedure. Most patients with FSHD have little to no decreased pulmonary function compared to unaffected patients and disease course is generally slow, with a normal life-expectancy [31–33, 56]. Therefore, most patients would have a greater overall benefit from a scapulothoracic arthrodesis as the range of motion and daily function is retained over time. Patients should be warned that both cross-body adduction and internal rotation behind the body will be limited post-operatively.

Intra-operatively, important considerations include how to position and prep the patient and where to anchor the scapula on the thoracic wall. Prepping and draping the entire upper extremity into the surgical field allows the surgeon to check pulses in the extremity to confirm that scapular stabilization has not affected the vascular supply to the upper extremity. Mackenzie et al. reported taking a patient back to the operating room for immediate revision after the patient was noted to have a cold upper extremity in the post-anesthesia recovery area [57]. Repositioning the scapula on the ribs resulted in immediate return of the radial pulse [57]. Including the extremity in the sterile field also allows the surgeon to range the arm after scapular stabilization to test the strength of the fixation. Most authors recommend attaching the scapula to the third through sixth or fourth through seventh ribs, in no more than 30° of external rotation. Preoperative evaluation can help the surgeon plan how to position the scapula on the thoracic wall to achieve optimal range of motion for the patient. Once the scapula is fixed to the ribs, it is recommended that the surgical field be filled with normal saline and that the anesthesia team initiate positive pressure ventilation to check for any leak in the pleura. If a leak is detected, a chest tube should be placed intra-operatively to prevent a pneumothorax post-operatively [49].

Although early reports of scapulopexy and scapulothoracic arthrodesis indicated that there were minimal complications with these procedures, more recent reports have shown that complication rates are higher than previously indicated. Goel et al. reported a 50% complication rate overall after scapulothoracic arthrodesis in 12 shoulders [49]. Intra-operative complications include pleural tear, pneumothorax, and hemothorax [49, 52, 53, 55, 58]. Brachial plexus palsy has been reported infrequently, but can be a devastating complication [47, 57, 59]. In scapulothoracic arthrodesis, non-union rates have been reported as frequently as 15–17% [47–49, 53, 55]. Most authors do not obtain routine post-operative CT scans on patients to evaluate for bony fusion, so the reported non-union rates are reflective of painful pseudoarthroses. It is possible that routine CT evaluation of patients at 6 or 12 months post-operatively would demonstrate a slightly higher nonunion rate than what is currently recorded in the literature. Rib and scapula fractures intra-operatively as well as rib stress fractures post-operatively have also been reported [53, 55, 58]. Post-operatively, painful hardware has been reported and studies have shown up to a 50% return to surgery rate for removal of hardware after arthrodesis is confirmed through imaging [49].

Early reports of both scapulopexy and scapulothoracic arthrodesis did not routinely analyze the effects that these procedures had on a patient's pulmonary function. However, more recent studies include the effects that these surgeries have on patients' pulmonary function tests immediately after the procedure and during follow-up. Studies show that there are usually mild losses in FEV1 and forced vital capacity after unilateral scapulothoracic arthrodesis, but more significant decline can be seen after bilateral surgeries [44, 47, 48, 50, 54, 55, 58]. However, there are isolated reports of significant decline in pulmonary function after unilateral surgeries [58].

Patients with FSHD do not generally require operative intervention for the lower extremities or the spine. If tibialis anterior and/or peroneal weakness develops, patients may develop a flexible equinus or equinovarus foot position. This usually responds well to bracing with ankle-foot orthoses. If the deformity becomes rigid, the patient could undergo an intramuscular lengthening [33, 56]. Scoliosis is rare in patients with facioscapulohumeral dystrophy. If a curve greater than 40–50° develops, it should be managed following the same principles that one would use to manage adolescent idiopathic scoliosis [56]. Patients often develop hyperlordosis and, if severe, this can be managed with an orthosis. However, an orthosis may interfere with the patient's ability to ambulate, as hyperlordosis allows the patient to compensate for progressive hip extensor weakness [56].

## Infantile Facioscapulohumeral Muscular Dystrophy

Infantile facioscapulohumeral muscular dystrophy (iFSHD) has become increasingly recognized as a related but distinct disease process over the past several decades [31, 32, 56, 60–63]. Although molecular evaluation has shown that the same gene is affected as in adolescent facioscapulohumeral dystrophy, the disease course is more rapid and clinically this mirrors more severe MDs, such as Duchenne [61]. Infants usually develop facial diplegia [62]. Children begin walking at a normal age, but they rapidly develop pelvic girdle weakness. Children can have a positive Gower's sign and demonstrate significant hip extensor weakness on exam. They develop marked, severe hyperlordosis and use their hands to help stabilize their hip extensors while standing and walking, which is a near pathognomonic sign of this disease [63]. An equinus foot position develops, usually as a compensatory measure for quadriceps and tibialis anterior weakness. Patients develop shoulder girdle weakness, but unlike their adolescent and adult counterparts, it is the pelvic girdle weakness that dictates treatment in these patients.

The overall treatment goal for patients with iFSHD is to preserve function. Although hyperlordosis is severe, these patients do not respond well to bracing and use of orthoses should be limited. The hyperlordosis is a compensatory development, meant to counter the severe hip extensor weakness in these patients. Correcting the hyperlordosis with a brace or with surgery can actually inhibit ambulation because the patient can no longer compensate for their pelvic girdle weakness [33, 63]. Similarly, the equinus foot position is also a compensatory measure. Most children respond well to ankle-foot orthoses or knee-ankle-foot orthoses, but on the rare occasion when a patient develops a rigid equinovarus foot position, an intramuscular lengthening could be considered [33, 63].

Most patients lose the ability to ambulate by the second or third decade [60–62]. If the hyperlordosis is severe at that point, one could consider either bracing or surgical intervention to improve the patient's ability to sit in a wheel chair [33]. The shoulder girdle weakness is typically not a limiting condition for these patients because their spine and lower extremity conditions tend to be more severe. If the shoulder girdle weakness does interfere significantly with daily function, scapular stabilization can be considered. Scapulopexy is favored over scapulorthoracic arthrodesis in these settings because it allows immediate shoulder range of motion, there is no post-operative immobilization, and the procedure has less of an effect on pulmonary function, which is significantly more limited in patients with infantile facioscapulohumeral dystrophy. Scapular stabilization is not routinely performed in these patients because their disease course is so rapid, and the patients lose function in their upper extremities so quickly that the surgical benefits would not outweigh surgical risks to make the procedure worthwhile [32].

## Limb-Girdle Muscular Dystrophy

Limb-girdle muscular dystrophy (LGMD) encompasses an increasing number of diseases that cause proximal muscle weakness, especially of the shoulders, pelvic region, and thighs. Due to the heterogeneity of this diagnosis, specific recommendations should be tailored to the genetically diagnosed disease. This section's brevity reflects the difficulty in recommending orthopaedic management for this group of diseases as they all present varying clinical phenotypes.

## Non-operative Management

LGMD is a general diagnosis that encompasses at least 16 genetically distinct disease processes [32]. As such, the manifestations of the disease can vary significantly from one patient to another, depending on the underlying genetic abnormality. Overall, symptoms and disease progression mimic that of BMD. Most treatment is supportive and includes physical therapy and orthoses to maximize muscle strength and prevent contracture formation [64, 65].

## Operative Management

Surgical indications are similar to those utilized for BMD [31]. Unlike patients with DMD, scoliosis does not develop in most patients with LGMD. Patients who do develop scoliosis also generally have mild curves that do not require surgical intervention [32, 33].

## References

1. Biggar WD, et al. Long-term benefits of deflazacort treatment for boys with Duchenne muscular dystrophy in their second decade. Neuromuscul Disord. 2006;16(4):249–55.
2. Bushby K, et al. Diagnosis and management of Duchenne muscular dystrophy, part 1: diagnosis, and pharmacological and psychosocial management. Lancet Neurol. 2010;9(1):77–93.
3. King WM, et al. Orthopedic outcomes of long-term daily corticosteroid treatment in Duchenne muscular dystrophy. Neurology. 2007;68(19):1607–13.
4. Lebel DE, et al. Glucocorticoid treatment for the prevention of scoliosis in children with Duchenne muscular dystrophy: long-term follow-up. J Bone Joint Surg Am. 2013;95(12): 1057–61.
5. Bothwell JE, et al. Vertebral fractures in boys with Duchenne muscular dystrophy. Clin Pediatr. 2003;42(4):353–6.
6. James KA, et al. Risk factors for first fractures among males with Duchenne or Becker muscular dystrophy. J Pediatr Orthop. 2014.
7. Pouwels S, et al. Risk of fracture in patients with muscular dystrophies. Osteoporos Int. 2014;25(2):509–18.
8. Main M, et al. Serial casting of the ankles in Duchenne muscular dystrophy: can it be an alternative to surgery? Neuromuscul Disord. 2007;17(3):227–30.
9. Bushby K, et al. Diagnosis and management of Duchenne muscular dystrophy, part 2: implementation of multidisciplinary care. Lancet Neurol. 2010;9(2):177–89.
10. Garralda ME, et al. Knee-ankle-foot orthosis in children with Duchenne muscular dystrophy: user views and adjustment. Eur J Paediatr Neurol. 2006;10(4):186–91.
11. Siegel IM. Maintenance of ambulation in Duchenne muscular dystrophy. The role of the orthopedic surgeon. Clin Pediatr. 1980;19(6):383–8.
12. Alemdaroglu I, et al. Different types of upper extremity exercise training in Duchenne muscular dystrophy: effects on functional performance, strength, endurance, and ambulation. Muscle Nerve. 2014.

13. Bartels B, et al. Upper limb function in adults with Duchenne muscular dystrophy. J Rehabil Med. 2011;43(9):770–5.
14. Mattar FL, Sobreira C. Hand weakness in Duchenne muscular dystrophy and its relation to physical disability. Neuromuscul Disord. 2008;18(3):193–8.
15. Arun R, Srinivas S, Mehdian SM. Scoliosis in Duchenne's muscular dystrophy: a changing trend in surgical management: a historical surgical outcome study comparing sublaminar, hybrid and pedicle screw instrumentation systems. Eur Spine J. 2010;19(3):376–83.
16. Hsu JD. The natural history of spine curvature progression in the nonambulatory Duchenne muscular dystrophy patient. Spine. 1983;8(7):771–5.
17. Karol LA. Scoliosis in patients with Duchenne muscular dystrophy. J Bone Joint Surg Am. 2007. 89 Suppl. 1:155–62.
18. Kurz LT, et al. Correlation of scoliosis and pulmonary function in Duchenne muscular dystrophy. J Pediatr Orthop. 1983;3(3):347–53.
19. Miller F, et al. Pulmonary function and scoliosis in Duchenne dystrophy. J Pediatr Orthop. 1988;8(2):133–7.
20. Shapiro F, et al. Progression of spinal deformity in wheelchair-dependent patients with Duchenne muscular dystrophy who are not treated with steroids: coronal plane (scoliosis) and sagittal plane (kyphosis, lordosis) deformity. Bone Joint J. 2014;96-B(1):100–5.
21. Gray B, Hsu JD, Furumasu J. Fractures caused by falling from a wheelchair in patients with neuromuscular disease. Dev Med Child Neurol. 1992;34(7):589–92.
22. Leitch KK, et al. Should foot surgery be performed for children with Duchenne muscular dystrophy? J Pediatr Orthop. 2005;25(1):95–7.
23. Scher DM, Mubarak SJ. Surgical prevention of foot deformity in patients with Duchenne muscular dystrophy. J Pediatr Orthop. 2002;22(3):384–91.
24. Yamashita T, et al. Prediction of progression of spinal deformity in Duchenne muscular dystrophy: a preliminary report. Spine. 2001;26(11):E223–6.
25. Alman BA, Kim HK. Pelvic obliquity after fusion of the spine in Duchenne muscular dystrophy. J Bone Joint Surg Br. 1999;81(5):821–4.
26. Bui T, Shapiro F. Posterior spinal fusion to sacrum in non-ambulatory hypotonic neuromuscular patients: sacral rod/bone graft onlay method. J Child Orthop. 2014;8(3):229–36.
27. Sengupta DK, et al. Pelvic or lumbar fixation for the surgical management of scoliosis in Duchenne muscular dystrophy. Spine. 2002;27(18):2072–9.
28. Duckworth AD, Mitchell MJ, Tsirikos AI. Incidence and risk factors for post-operative complications after scoliosis surgery in patients with Duchenne muscular dystrophy: a comparison with other neuromuscular conditions. Bone Joint J. 2014;96-B(7):943–9.
29. Ramirez N, et al. Complications after posterior spinal fusion in Duchenne's muscular dystrophy. J Pediatr Orthop. 1997;17(1):109–14.
30. Johnsen SD. Prednisone therapy in Becker's muscular dystrophy. J Child Neurol. 2001;16(11):870–1.
31. Lovell WW, Weinstein SL, Flynn JM. Lovell and Winter's pediatric orthopaedics. 7th ed. Philadelphia: Wolters Kluwer Health/Lippincott Williams & Wilkins; 2014.
32. Herring JA, Tachdjian MO. Texas Scottish Rite Hospital for Children. Tachdjian's pediatric orthopaedics. 4th ed. Philadelphia: Saunders/Elsevier; 2008.
33. Shapiro F, Specht L. The diagnosis and orthopaedic treatment of inherited muscular diseases of childhood. J Bone Joint Surg Am. 1993;75(3):439–54.
34. Daher YH, Lonstein JE, Winter RB, Bradford DS. Spinal deformities in patients with muscular dystrophy other than Duchenne. A review of 11 patients having surgical treatment. Spine. 1985;10(7):614–7.
35. Andersen SP, Sveen ML, Hansen RS, et al. Creatine kinase response to high-intensity aerobic exercise in adult-onset muscular dystrophy. Muscle Nerve. 2013;48(6):897–901.
36. Olsen DB, Orngreen MC, Vissing J. Aerobic training improves exercise performance in facioscapulohumeral muscular dystrophy. Neurology. 2005;64(6):1064–6.

37. Bakhtiary AH, Phoenix J, Edwards RH, Frostick SP. The effect of motor learning in facioscapulohumeral muscular dystrophy patients. Eur J Appl Physiol. 2000;83(6):551–8.
38. Pasotti S, Magnani B, Longa E, et al. An integrated approach in a case of facioscapulohumeral dystrophy. BMC Musculoskelet Disord. 2014;15:155.
39. D'Antona G, Ragni M, Cardile A, et al. Branched-chain amino acid supplementation promotes survival and supports cardiac and skeletal muscle mitochondrial biogenesis in middle-aged mice. Cell Metab. 2010;12(4):362–72.
40. Tarnopolsky M, Zimmer A, Paikin J, et al. Creatine monohydrate and conjugated linoleic acid improve strength and body composition following resistance exercise in older adults. PLoS One. 2007;2(10):e991.
41. Tarnopolsky MA. Creatine as a therapeutic strategy for myopathies. Amino Acids. 2011;40(5):1397–407.
42. Kissel JT, McDermott MP, Natarajan R, et al. Pilot trial of albuterol in facioscapulohumeral muscular dystrophy. FSH-DY Group. Neurology. 1998;50(5):1402–6.
43. Kissel JT, McDermott MP, Mendell JR, et al. Randomized, double-blind, placebo-controlled trial of albuterol in facioscapulohumeral dystrophy. Neurology. 2001;57(8):1434–40.
44. Giannini S, Ceccarelli F, Faldini C, Pagkrati S, Merlini L. Scapulopexy of winged scapula secondary to facioscapulohumeral muscular dystrophy. Clin Orthop Relat Res. 2006;449:288–94.
45. Ketenjian AY. Scapulocostal stabilization for scapular winging in facioscapulohumeral muscular dystrophy. J Bone Joint Surg Am. 1978;60(4):476–80.
46. Bunch WH, Siegel IM. Scapulothoracic arthrodesis in facioscapulohumeral muscular dystrophy. Review of seventeen procedures with three to twenty-one-year follow-up. J Bone Joint Surg Am. 1993;75(3):372–6.
47. Cooney AD, Gill I, Stuart PR. The outcome of scapulothoracic arthrodesis using cerclage wires, plates, and allograft for facioscapulohumeral dystrophy. J Shoulder Elbow Surg. 2014;23(1):e8–13.
48. Demirhan M, Uysal O, Atalar AC, Kilicoglu O, Serdaroglu P. Scapulothoracic arthrodesis in facioscapulohumeral dystrophy with multifilament cable. Clin Orthop Relat Res. 2009;467(8):2090–7.
49. Goel DP, Romanowski JR, Shi LL, Warner JJ. Scapulothoracic fusion: outcomes and complications. J Shoulder Elbow Surg. 2014;23(4):542–7.
50. Jakab E, Gledhill RB. Simplified technique for scapulocostal fusion in facioscapulohumeral dystrophy. J Pediatr Orthop. 1993;13(6):749–51.
51. Kocialkowski A, Frostick SP, Wallace WA. One-stage bilateral thoracoscapular fusion using allografts. A case report. Clin Orthop Relat Res. 1991;273:264–7.
52. Krishnan SG, Hawkins RJ, Michelotti JD, Litchfield R, Willis RB, Kim YK. Scapulothoracic arthrodesis: indications, technique, and results. Clin Orthop Relat Res. 2005;435:126–33.
53. Letournel E, Fardeau M, Lytle JO, Serrault M, Gosselin RA. Scapulothoracic arthrodesis for patients who have facioscapulohumeral muscular dystrophy. J Bone Joint Surg Am. 1990;72(1):78–84.
54. Rhee YG, Ha JH. Long-term results of scapulothoracic arthrodesis of facioscapulohumeral muscular dystrophy. J Shoulder Elbow Surg. 2006;15(4):445–50.
55. Twyman RS, Harper GD, Edgar MA. Thoracoscapular fusion in facioscapulohumeral dystrophy: clinical review of a new surgical method. J Shoulder Elbow Surg. 1996;5(3):201–5.
56. Birch JG. Orthopedic management of neuromuscular disorders in children. Semin Pediatr Neurol. 1998;5(2):78–91.
57. Mackenzie WG, Riddle EC, Earley JL, Sawatzky BJ. A neurovascular complication after scapulothoracic arthrodesis. Clin Orthop Relat Res. 2003;408:157–61.
58. Berne D, Laude F, Laporte C, Fardeau M, Saillant G. Scapulothoracic arthrodesis in facioscapulohumeral muscular dystrophy. Clin Orthop Relat Res. 2003;409:106–13.
59. Wolfe GI, Young PK, Nations SP, Burkhead WZ, McVey AL, Barohn RJ. Brachial plexopathy following thoracoscapular fusion in facioscapulohumeral muscular dystrophy. Neurology. 2005;64(3):572–3.

60. Bailey RO, Marzulo DC, Hans MB. Infantile facioscapulohumeral muscular dystrophy: new observations. Acta Neurol Scand. 1986;74(1):51–8.
61. Brouwer OF, Padberg GW, Wijmenga C, Frants RR. Facioscapulohumeral muscular dystrophy in early childhood. Arch Neurol. 1994;51(4):387–94.
62. Korf BR, Bresnan MJ, Shapiro F, Sotrel A, Abroms IF. Facioscapulohumeral dystrophy presenting in infancy with facial diplegia and sensorineural deafness. Ann Neurol. 1985;17(5): 513–6.
63. Shapiro F, Specht L, Korf BR. Locomotor problems in infantile facioscapulohumeral muscular dystrophy. Retrospective study of 9 patients. Acta Orthop Scand. 1991;62(4):367–71.
64. Narayanaswami P, Weiss M, Selcen D, et al. Evidence-based guideline summary: diagnosis and treatment of limb-girdle and distal dystrophies: report of the guideline development subcommittee of the American Academy of Neurology and the practice issues review panel of the American Association of Neuromuscular & Electrodiagnostic Medicine. Neurology. 2014; 83(16):1453–63.
65. Wicklund MP, Kissel JT. The limb-girdle muscular dystrophies. Neurol Clin. 2014;32(3):729–49. 3.

# Chapter 10
# Global Regulatory Landscape

Raymond A. Huml

## Introduction

To address the best way to study potential treatments for muscular dystrophy (MD), the International Conference on Harmonization (ICH) communities have responded by issuing draft guidance in Europe, although not as fully or completely as patients, caregivers, or healthcare providers would like. The situation has similarities to that for biosimilars, where the European Union is ahead of the U.S. with regard to specific regulatory guidance. The European Medicines Agency (EMA) issued a concept paper in 2011 and, in early 2013, draft guidance for treatments related to DMD and BMD.

As of April 17, 2015, there are no disease-modifying products approved for the treatment of MD, but that situation may soon change. On May 23, 2014, reversing an earlier rejection, the EU Committee for Medicinal Products for Human Use (CHMP) recommended early (conditional) approval for PTC Therapeutics' ataluren (Translarna™), a potential treatment for DMD. CHMP initially refused approval because the product failed to significantly improve DMD patients' scores on a six-minute walk test compared with placebo. During re-examination, the CHMP took the view that there was some evidence of effectiveness when the drug was used at a dose of 40 mg/kg/day and that the mechanism of action for this effectiveness was plausible [1, 2].

If the European Commission supports this decision (and it usually follows the advice of the CHMP), ataluren would be the first product approved, albeit conditionally, for MD—until the final Phase III data are available. If the clinical data for that trial are robust, the conditional approval can be expected to turn into full approval.

R.A. Huml, M.S., D.V.M., R.A.C. (✉)
Biosimilars Center of Excellence, Quintiles Inc., 4820 Emperor Boulevard,
Durham, NC 27703, USA
e-mail: raymond.huml@quintiles.com

© Springer International Publishing Switzerland 2015
R.A. Huml (ed.), *Muscular Dystrophy*, DOI 10.1007/978-3-319-17362-7_10

The U.S., on the other hand, appears to be relying on programs already in place to address the issues related to the potential treatment of MD, and no MD products have been recommended for approval. In 2013, when the U.S. Food and Drug Administration (FDA) addressed concerns from patient advocacy groups such as the Muscular Dystrophy Association (MDA), it cited existing programs to address the lack of specific MD regulatory guidance in the U.S. Programs specifically discussed included Fast Track Designation, Breakthrough Therapy Designation, Accelerated Approval, and Priority Review [3].

The FDA's reluctance to develop specific guidelines for MD research is, apparently, not acceptable to caregiver and patient communities. Take for example, Parent Project Muscular Dystrophy (PPMD), which, in conjunction with other stakeholders, submitted the first-ever patient advocacy-initiated draft guidance to the FDA to help accelerate development and review of potential treatments for DMD [4].

This chapter provides an overview of the budding regulatory landscape for the treatment of MD in the EU and argues for more-detailed U.S. FDA guidance, even if it means reaching out to advocacy groups to include regulatory guidance for non-Duchenne types of MD.

## EU Regulatory Guidance

New perspectives have emerged for future therapeutic options in DMD and BMD. The increasing numbers of clinical trials that recruit the rather small number of patients for these progressive disorders have raised several issues, including their study design, the choice of appropriate efficacy endpoints in general, and the definition of reliable surrogate outcome measures, as well as the need for subgroup analyses with respect to this heterogeneous patient population and the duration of the trials (e.g., long-term treatment goals).

As most cases of DMD have an onset in early childhood, while the onset of BMD covers a broader age spectrum, specific difficulties have been identified that pertain to diagnostic criteria, age- and stage-related clinical relevance, and various safety aspects.

The EU is ahead of other ICH regions regarding issuance of regulatory guidance for treatments for MD. For example, EMA published a draft guideline entitled *Guideline on the Clinical Investigation of Medicinal Products for the Treatment of Duchenne and Becker Muscular Dystrophy* [5] that has been adopted by the CHMP and was released on February 21, 2013.

The draft guideline was the direct result of an EMA-issued concept paper entitled, *Concept Paper on the Need for a Guideline on the Treatment of Duchenne and Becker Muscular Dystrophy*, which was released for consultation on June 23, 2011 [6].

An overview of regulatory guidance addressing MD-specific drug development issued by EMA is provided in Table 10.1.

The draft version of the guideline was intended to provide guidance for the evaluation of medicinal products in the treatment of these diseases, including study

**Table 10.1** EMA-issued regulatory guidance specifically for the treatment of MD

| Document | Reference number | Publication date |
|---|---|---|
| Concept paper on the need for a guideline on the treatment of Duchenne and Becker muscular dystrophy | EMA/CHMP/CNSWP/236981/2011 | – Adoption by CHMP for release for consultation June 23, 2011 |
| | | – End of consultation (deadline for comments) September 30, 2011 |
| (Draft) guideline on the clinical investigation of medicinal products for the treatment of Duchenne and Becker muscular dystrophy | EMA/CHMP/236981/2011 | – Adoption by CHMP for release for consultation February 21, 2013 |
| | | – End of consultation (deadline for comments) August 31, 2013 |

design, choice of appropriate efficacy endpoints, and definition of reliable surrogate outcome measures.

The scope of the guideline is limited to DMD, the most severe form of MD, and the milder version, BMD. Other neuromuscular diseases, such as FSHD, are currently outside the scope of this guideline.

Highlights of the document are described below. These include factors related to study design:

1. Outcomes that reflect improvement in symptoms and in disability in affected patients (maintenance of muscle strength and function, prevention of damage to non-muscular target organs [such as the lung, heart, and eyes], orthopedic corrections, and physiotherapeutic interventions).
2. In confirmatory trials, the efficacy and safety of the product should be studied in the full range of patients that the investigational product is intended to treat.
3. Confirmatory trials to show symptom or disability improvement should be randomized, double-blind, parallel group, and possibly placebo-controlled.
4. Trials investigating symptomatic treatment should last at least three months; trials to show an improvement in disability, at least six months.

The document also examines the choice of appropriate efficacy endpoints:

1. For patients without a confirmed genetic diagnosis, a combination of clinical symptoms, family history, elevated creatine kinase (CK) concentration, magnetic resonance imaging (MRI), and muscle biopsy is considered sufficient for a diagnosis, but it is not sufficient for inclusion in clinical trials in which potential medicinal products targeting certain type of genetic defects are investigated.
2. Efficacy: the objectives of the study should be well-defined according to the expected stage- and age-related improvement in certain types of symptom domains (e.g., walking, daily functioning, maintaining ambulant state, use of upper limb in non-ambulant subjects, and overall survival).
3. Muscle strength should be evaluated by clinical assessment using a validated tool.

The document also provides a definition of reliable surrogate outcome measures:

1. Modifications of the natural course of the disease (which causes continued muscular weakness) or increasing survival (clinically, a sustained effect on disability progression has to be shown).
2. Improvement in motor function could be achieved by correcting or counteracting the underlying genetic defect, by increasing muscle growth and regeneration, or by modulating inflammatory responses.

## U.S. Regulatory Guidance

Although no formal guidance related to treatments for MD has been issued in the U.S. (at the time this chapter was written), several notable milestones have been reached, edging the U.S. closer to releasing formal regulatory guidance. Consider the following:

Six FDA officers published an article addressing issues associated with DMD drug development. See the paper by McNeil and colleagues for additional details [7].

FDA's Office of Orphan Products Development (OOPD) has provided grant funding to support two studies of products to treat DMD and has granted orphan designation to 15 products for the treatment of DMD [8].

A webinar aimed at increasing dialogue between patient advocacy groups and FDA and entitled, "Accelerated Approval–Duchenne Disease," was presented by Robert Temple, MD, deputy center director for Clinical Science, Center for Drug Evaluation and Research, on February 20, 2013 [9]. Temple cited 21 CFR 312.80 (Subpart E) of 1988 Investigational New Drug (IND) registration for "serious and life-threatening diseases" and then discussed four pathways that could be leveraged for the study of treatments for MD: (1) Fast Track Designation, (2) Breakthrough Therapy Designation, (3) Accelerated Approval, and (4) Priority Review. These four pathways, it should be noted, are not specific for MD.

Examples of FDA's use of existing pathways over the last three years include granting orphan drug status to Acceleron Pharma's ACE-031 (August 2010) [10] and Breakthrough Therapy Designation to Prosensa for drisapersen (June 2013) [11]. Prosensa regained the rights to drisapersen from GSK in January 2014 [12].

However, even though the FDA has not yet issued specific guidance for MD treatments, the agency appears to be willing to accept assistance from others—especially given the rarity of the disease and paucity of clinical trial data collected to date. In a letter dated June 25, 2014, from Pat Long, President of PPMD, to FDA's Dr. Janet Woodcock, the group announced that it had met as a forum with the FDA on December 12, 2013 and concluded with an agreement that the Duchenne community, led by the PPMD, would develop the first draft guidance on Duchenne for industry.

The draft guidance, titled, *Guidance for Industry: Duchenne Muscular Dystrophy, Developing Drugs for Treatment over the Spectrum of Disease,* is unprecedented since, to the author's knowledge, the FDA has not, to date, accepted input from advocacy groups with the goal of issuing guidance to industry. Indeed, in a PR Newswire news release titled, "First-Ever Patient Initiated 'Guidance for Industry' for Duchenne Muscular Dystrophy," the PPMD President is quoted as saying: "This landmark guidance represents a major milestone for the Duchenne community and may open the way for other rare disease groups to incorporate the patient perspective in a well-documented and quantifiable way." In the panel on Page 1 of the guidance, the first line states, "This draft guidance represents the first FDA guidance initially composed by a disease community, with input from industry, sponsors, academia and the DMD patient community."

Written in a form similar to historical draft FDA guidances, the DMD document was written to help accelerate the development and review of potential therapies for Duchenne MD.

As acknowledged by the members and subcommittees who wrote the Guidance for Industry, it is possible that the Agency may choose not to formally adopt all or part of the proposed guidance in the future. However, since there is no other official guidance in the U.S. and some of the DMD-specific material is already covered in the EU draft guidance, a summary of the PPMD document is highlighted below, noting the sections that may have significance and relevance for the other types of MD.

## PPMD/U.S. Issued Guidance for Industry

Caregiver tolerance to risk "does not mean flexibility with regard to whether a trial's findings are statistically significant," PPMD said in its cover letter to the guidance [13].

> Rather, the flexibility we are seeking may concern where the line is drawn as to whether an intermediate clinical endpoint is clinically meaningful, whether post-hoc analyses can support an NDA [New Drug Application] or whether a less-than-precise biomarker is reasonably likely to produce clinical benefit.
>
> "Families affected by Duchenne often feel as if the FDA is an untouchable and unreachable group of professionals tasked with making critical decisions on potential drugs," the letter states. "Consequently, the community has been advocating that the FDA be more flexible in its review of rare and progressive diseases like Duchenne and to decrease the time and cost of conducting those trials for companies engaged in or considering trials for potential therapies for Duchenne... given some of the recent delays."

It will be interesting to see the potential effect of the PPMD guidance should an NDA for Sarepta's eteplirsen for Duchenne MD be submitted to FDA, a step planned for mid 2015 [14].

The proposed guidance is divided into the following areas aimed at overcoming challenges in trial design and implementation:

- Benefit–Risk Assessment: This section takes the position that clinical trial sponsors should engage with the patient advocacy community from the start of drug development to understand "that meaningful benefit risk tolerance and acceptable trade-offs may vary across clinical subtypes, across disease progression status, or as a consequence of preference heterogeneity across patients, parents and caregivers." A recent survey published in *Clinical Therapeutics* [15] provides new insights into caregiver perspectives on benefits and risks of emerging therapies for DMD, the most common form of the disease. The survey, carried out by researchers from the PPMD and Johns Hopkins Bloomberg School of Public Health, found that "caregivers were willing to accept a serious risk when balanced with a noncurative treatment, even absent improvement in life span." A total of 119 DMD caregivers completed the online survey, which used best–worst scaling. Six relevant and understandable attributes describing potential benefits and risks of emerging DMD therapies were identified through engagement with advocates, clinicians, pharmaceutical companies, academic centers, and other stakeholders. The attributes were: muscle function, life span, knowledge about the drug, nausea, risk of bleeds, and risk of arrhythmia. Treatment effect on muscle function was rated as the most important experimental attribute (28.7%), followed by risk of heart arrhythmia (22.4%) and risk of bleeding (21.2%). Having additional post-approval data was relatively the least important attribute (2.3%). The authors emphasized that "these preferences should inform the FDA's benefit–risk assessment of emerging DMD therapies."

- Diagnosis: This section refers sponsors to guidance from the American Academy of Pediatrics on a diagnostic algorithm. It notes the characteristic diagnostic delay with DMD and the importance of genetic analysis, including access to genetic testing.
- Natural History: This characterizes the clinical course of DMD, including details of scientific consensus on tools, instruments, and outcome measures.
- Clinical Trial Designs, Outcome Measures, and Considerations: This section underscores the need for trials to include patients of all ages and disease stages where possible.
- Biomarkers: This examines the role of biomarkers in DMD clinical trials, including:

  - Muscle Biopsy-Based Biomarkers: Considerations when performing muscle biopsies include the ethical imperative to perform them only when needed and to take precautions to ensure usable specimens. This section includes an examination of international efforts to standardize methodologies and emerging technologies.
  - Non-Muscle Biopsy-Based Biomarkers: This explores the potential for noninvasive imaging techniques to replace biopsies, such as MRI/MRS skeletal muscle imaging, with the ultimate goal of using these as a surrogate endpoint for treatment trials.

Just as important for other types of MDs, the cover letter notes that there are critical unmet medical needs across the entire spectrum of the disease—at all ages, stages, and in each subpopulation.

The cover letter notes the importance of time to diagnosis, which for DMD, can take parents years to get a diagnosis for their child. They note that this reduces the number of young patients who could be enrolled in clinical trials at a stage of the disease when they might be able to most likely benefit and recommend routine newborn screening to help resolve this issue.

Specific for clinical trials, and important for patients with other types of MD, the cover letter highlights several important clinical trial considerations, highlighted below:

- Include all ages to whatever degree possible.
- Move away from placebo-controlled trials or use trial designs that minimize exposure to placebo.
- Sponsors to address co-morbid conditions which may become exacerbated if new therapies do help prolong life and function.
- Flexibility in the interpretation of post-hoc statistical analysis, especially for rare diseases.
- Provide families with access to individual data (for their child/patient).
- Sponsors are expected to provide Informed Consent that covers:

  - Whether the company has a policy on pre-approval compassionate use (and/ or plans for expanded access programs) and if one child with MD in a family has access to the treatment, to allow other family members access as well.
  - What that policy is.
  - What the expectation is about expanding into an extension phase of the study after a trial is done and if there are positive results.

- Sponsors are encouraged to make trials more patient-friendly—especially for non-ambulatory patients with limited mobility—including trials or parts of trials closer to home.

## Specific Notes from the PPMD Guidance Applicable to All Types of MD

The PPMD Guidance includes the following notes that apply to all types of MD:

- DMD, like other types of MD, has known inherited features and the existence of de novo mutations which cause the phenotype of the disease.
- DMD, like other types of MD, is rare, and advancement and new treatments depends on patient advocacy groups to represent the views of its patients and caregivers.
- At the time of writing, there are no MD-specific therapies approved in the U.S.
- Need to incorporate the perspectives of patients and their families via conjoint analysis—a broad class of methods that includes discrete-choice experiments.
- Sponsors should explore risk-mitigation strategies and patient/caregiver preferences for these strategies.
- Sponsors should anticipate that appraisals of benefit/risk will change over time due to disease and non-disease-related factors and available treatment options.

- The certainty of disease progression without treatment should be included as a compelling harm in the benefit–risk assessment.
- Patients screened with older techniques may need to be re-tested in order to more accurately characterize their mutations (as entry criteria for potential clinical trials).
- Sponsors should be aware that a molecular diagnosis is not the same as a clinical diagnosis and does not, with a 100% certainty, determine phenotype.
- The natural history of certain types of MD is much better characterized today than 10–20 years ago, as a consequence of patient registries, natural history studies, and data drawn from the placebo arms of industry trials.
- After MD patients can no longer walk, there is continued muscular deterioration throughout the upper and lower limbs, and skeletal deformities such as limb contractures and spine deformity may become problematic.
- Maintaining computer access is a critical quality of life concern.
- Most lower limb and upper limb contractures occur subsequent to the loss of ambulation.
- Many development scales require formal training and certification on the part of the clinical investigator.
- "Time to run/walk 10 m" is predictive of future loss of ambulation.
- The six minute walk test has been the most commonly used primary outcome measure in DMD clinical development programs.
- MRI is the modality of choice when high resolution/high contrast images of skeletal tissue are demanded. MRI is a non-ionizing/noninvasive technique.

## Heterogeneity in Disease Progression

Muscle disease progression, as noted elsewhere, is variable, even within families. To address these differences, the following suggestions were made to account for heterogeneity in disease progression:

- The goal of therapeutics in MD is to slow or stabilize disease progression in comparison to that expected by natural history.
- Some variability in future progression is explained on the basis of disease severity, stage of disease, and known natural history.
- Sponsors should take care to prevent an imbalance in the ages of study participants, which can introduce substantial variability into a trial.
- Control and treatment arms in clinical trials should be appropriately matched by age and functional status.
- Clinical trials of treatments that are not mutation-specific should collect appropriate samples for full genetic analysis.
- Need to establish adequate, reliable, and well-matched natural history controls to account for known causes in variability.

## Treatment Effects by Muscle Group

Treatment effects may vary by muscle group depending upon (1) the stage of disease, (2) the differential rate of progression of each muscle group in that stage, (3) the muscle fiber type, (4) the drug's mechanism of action, (5) the bio-distribution of the drug to different tissues and muscle fiber types, (6) the route of administration, and (7) the medical addressability of the disease itself—there may be a point where a muscle has deteriorated beyond the possibility of responding to therapy.

## Gaps in Data

Some notable gaps in performing clinical DMD clinical trials were highlighted, which may have ramifications for treatments for other types of MD, and include the following:

- At present, there is no single instrument that can measure clinical outcomes and is equally sensitive to change across the entire spectrum of DMD over the course of a 6–18 months study.
- The non-ambulant population needs validated outcome measures for future therapeutic trials.
- A number of patient-reported outcomes (PROs) in DMD have been used or are being evaluated, but none has been validated.
- Although the PPMD group would like to move away from placebo-controlled trials, in favor of natural history matched controls, the document mentions that "the likelihood for results that are difficult to interpret with using natural history controls is substantially greater than in randomized placebo controlled trials."
- All biomarkers for use in DMD trials (as mentioned in the guidance) are exploratory.

## Summary

With scientific and clinical advances, it is becoming more commercially desirable to investigate new treatments for MD. Since MD can exist in many forms and manifests itself in a heterogenous manner, new treatments have been elusive. Because MD can be life threatening, new treatments, especially those that can be disease modifying (slowing down or halting disease progression) or curative (restoring normal function), are desperately needed.

Progress is being made toward the issuance of regulatory guidance in ICH countries for drug development for certain types of MD. The EU leads the pack with draft guidance issued in 2013 for DMD and BMD. While still early days, it appears that additional guidance will eventually be issued for the other forms of MD in order to de-risk programs and make it easier for drug developers to invest in new treatments.

At present, it appears the U.S. is taking a conservative approach, relying on its current programs that can be tweaked to help sponsors of products for the treatment of MD launch these on the U.S. market, but in an unprecedented move, solicited the first-ever draft guidance for industry written on behalf of a patient advocacy group with a focus on DMD. As acknowledged by the members and subcommittees who wrote the (DMD specific) Guidance for Industry, it is possible that the Agency may choose not to formally adopt all or part of the proposed guidance in the future. Since there is no other official guidance in the U.S., the PPMD document serves as a precedent for other types of MDs.

This trend for increasing collaboration between FDA and outside groups is confirmed in a July 2014 agency report titled, *Complex Issues in Developing Drugs and Biological Products for Rare Diseases and Accelerating the Development of Therapies for Pediatric Rare Diseases* [16]. The report covers MD from the perspective of available biomarkers and clinical outcome assessments [17]. It states FDA is working with external stakeholders to further develop the use of dystrophin as a biomarker for use in clinical trials of children with DMD.

It is unclear when or if U.S. guidance for the other forms of MD will be issued or if other patient advocacy groups will promulgate guidance in conjunction with the FDA.

Lack of formal U.S. guidance will add risk to sponsors' clinical drug development programs for the treatment of MD in the U.S. and may act as a disincentive to investment in potential new treatments. If adopted, the PPMD draft guidance could represent a step forward in de-risking this area for sponsors. The PPMD document also serves as a precedent for other groups as its contents, in common with those of the EU-sponsored guidance, overlap with other types of MD.

# References

1. PTC Therapeutics Website. PTC therapeutics receives positive opinion from CHMP for Translarna™ (Ataluren). 2014. http://ir.ptcbio.com/releasedetail.cfm?ReleaseID=850246. Accessed 9 July 2014.
2. Garde D. PTC soars as EU changes its tune on the DMD-treating ataluren. Fierce Biotech. http://www.fiercebiotech.com/story/ptc-soars-eu-changes-its-tune-dmd-treating-ataluren/2014-05-23. Accessed 9 Dec 2014.
3. Temple RJ. Accelerated approval, Duchenne muscular dystrophy webinar. http://support.cure-duchenne.org/site/PageNavigator/FDAWebinar.html. Accessed 19 Dec 2013.
4. First-ever patient-initiated "Guidance for Industry" for Duchenne muscular dystrophy submitted to FDA, PR Newswire. 2014. http://www.marketwatch.com/story/first-ever-patient-initiated-guidance-for-industry-for-duchenne-muscular-dystrophy-submitted-to-fda-2014-06-25. Accessed 5 July 2014.
5. Guideline on the clinical investigation of medicinal products for the treatment of Duchenne and Becker muscular dystrophy. European Medicines Agency website. http://www.ema.

europa.eu/docs/en_GB/document_library/Scientific_guideline/2013/03/WC500139508.pdf. Accessed 25 Oct 2013.

6. Concept paper on the need for a guideline on the treatment of Duchenne and Becker muscular dystrophy. European Medicines Agency website. http://www.ema.europa.eu/docs/en_GB/document_library/Scientific_guideline/2011/07/WC500108442.pdf. Accessed 25 Oct 2013.

7. McNeil DE, Davis C, Jillapalli D, Targum S, Durmowicz A, Cote TR. Duchenne muscular dystrophy: drug development and regulatory considerations. FDA Office of Orphan Product Development and Office of New Drugs. 2010 Wiley Periodicals; Published online in Wiley InterScience. http://onlinelibrary.wiley.com/doi/10.1002/mus.21623/full. Accessed 19 Dec 2013.

8. Duchenne's muscular dystrophy: Charlie's story at http://www.youtube.com/watch?v=4SL_TkGF25c. Accessed 19 Dec 2013.

9. Op cit 3.

10. Kotok A. Science and Enterprise, FDA Grants Orphan Status for Neuromuscular Drug. 2010. http://sciencebusiness.technewslit.com/?p=587. Accessed 19 Dec 2013.

11. Sherry C. Muscular dystrophy drug raises superiority issues in breakthrough path. 2013. http://jettfoundation.org/uncategorized/muscular-dystrophy-drug-raises-superiority-issues-in-breakthrough-path/. Accessed 19 Dec 2013.

12. Press release, 13 Jan 2014: Prosensa regains rights to drisapersen from GSK and retains rights to all other programmes for the treatment of Duchenne muscular dystrophy (DMD). http://www.gsk.com/media/press-releases/2014/prosensa-regains-rights-to-drisapersen-from-gsk-and-retains-righ.html. Accessed 10 Dec 2014.

13. Duchenne Community Imperatives and Cover Letter—Draft Guidance on Duchenne. 2014. Accessed 5 Aug 2014.

14. McCarthy E. Sarepta therapeutics sees setback in Eteplirsen drug application. Wall Street J. 2014. http://www.marketwatch.com/story/sarepta-therapuetics-sees-setback-in-eteplirsen-drug-applicaiton-2014-10-27-8103598. Accessed 9 Dec 2014.

15. Peay HL, Hollin I, Fischer R, Bridges JFB. A community-engaged approach to quantifying caregiver preferences for the benefits and risks of emerging therapies for Duchenne muscular dystrophy. Clin Ther. 2014;36:624–37.

16. U.S. Department of Health and Human Services, Food and Drug Administration. Report: complex issues in developing drugs and biological products for rare diseases and accelerating the development of therapies for pediatric rare diseases. 2014. http://www.fda.gov/downloads/RegulatoryInformation/Legislation/FederalFoodDrugandCosmeticActFDCAct/SignificantAmendmentstotheFDCAct/FDASIA/UCM404104.pdf. Accessed 22 July 2014.

17. Varond AJ. FDA releases report on rare diseases and accelerating the development of therapies for pediatric rare diseases. FDA Law Blog. 2014. http://www.fdalawblog.net/fda_law_blog_hyman_phelps/2014/07/fda-releases-report-on-rare-diseases-and-accelerating-the-development-of-therapies-for-pediatric-rar.html. Accessed 22 July 2014.

# Further Reading

Huml RA. Muscular dystrophy treatments: European and U.S. Regulatory Study Landscapes, RAPS regulatory focus, 6 p. Electronically posted to the RAPS website on 7 Jan 2014.

Huml RA. Filling a regulatory void: patient advocates submit guidance for Duchenne muscular dystrophy. RAPS regulatory focus, 5 p. Electronically posted to the RAPS website on 7 Aug 2014.

# Chapter 11
# Key Challenges to the Approval of Products to Treat Patients with Muscular Dystrophy

Raymond A. Huml

## Introduction

Although the first product for muscular dystrophy (MD) has been tentatively approved in Europe (for DMD), significant hurdles—including the identification of patients for clinical trials and the need to better understand the natural history of disease progression—remain to gaining regulatory approval of products to treat all patients with MD. Unfortunately, no MD products have yet been approved in the U.S.

The most progress has been made in DMD/BMD and the promulgation of regulatory guidance started in the EU in 2011. Regulatory advice is available in the EU for sponsors and investors in DMD/BMD clinical trials, which may help sponsors of products to treat other types of MD in the U.S. The U.S. is currently relying on programs already in place to advance products for rare diseases, including MD, and, in an unprecedented move, the FDA encouraged a patient advocacy group to submit draft guidance to help guide sponsors of MD products and decrease the risks associated with MD drug development.

Despite the challenges, substantial progress has been made and there are a number of late stage candidates in clinical development primarily for DMD (see Chapter 12 for a discussion of pharmaceutical products as potential treatments for patient with MD). Much more work is desperately needed to address the other eight types of MD.

Many people are not aware that MD is actually a group of diseases with different clinical manifestations and marked variance in progression, even within families and between siblings. The author has met multiple physicians and residents who have never seen a patient with FSHD or have only ever seen one or just a few patients with some type of MD. In addition, most of the types of MDs (e.g., oculopharyngeal MD

R.A. Huml, M.S., D.V.M., R.A.C. (✉)
Biosimilars Center of Excellence, Quintiles Inc., 4820 Emperor Boulevard,
Durham, NC 27703, USA
e-mail: raymond.huml@quintiles.com

and facioscapulohumeral MD) have very difficult names to pronounce and generally require an explanation to other family members, as well as healthcare providers (e.g., physician assistants), diagnostic technicians (e.g., x-ray technicians), and caregivers.

This lack of education and clinical awareness makes it difficult to discuss, much less manage, some of the risks associated with the clinical development and the capital required to develop products for the treatment of MD. This book is one small step towards narrowing this awareness gap.

The key challenges associated with the approval of products to treat patients with MD revolve around the science, which translates into therapeutic targets, and later to animal models of disease, and then to clinical trials in humans.

Natural history studies are required to understand the progression of the disease in groups or individuals with the disease. Once a long time-frame has been studied (e.g., >20 years), one can get an idea of the progression seen in a group of patients with a particular type of MD. Scientists who deem it unethical to study patients with MD using a placebo comparator arm (in case the drug is effective) may wish to study an investigational drug vs. the natural history progression to understand if disease progress is delayed or halted (by a disease-modifying therapy) or even better, reversed (a cure). Natural history studies are slowly being accomplished for MD types such as DMD and BMD, but less so for other types of MD. See Chapter 12 for additional details.

As the properties of an investigational drug become better known—usually through laboratory and animal experiments (during the preclinical phase of drug development)—scientists can develop and test theories to see if they can alter (upregulate, downregulate, or block) a biochemical pathway that might influence the disease in humans.

This chapter will begin with a discussion of two recently approved FDA documents (see Table 11.1), which provide the greatest amount of insight into MD drug development in the U.S., and end with a discussion of other considerations not included in the two regulatory documents. Interested readers (patients, caregivers, investors, drug developers) are encouraged to read both FDA documents in their entirety. One document, focused on rare diseases, was produced as a requirement of the FDA Safety and Innovation Act (Section 510 and PDUFA Performance Goals

**Table 11.1** Key FDA documents providing insights into MD clinical drug development in the U.S.

| Name of document | Date released |
| --- | --- |
| *Report: complex issues in developing drugs and biological products for rare diseases and accelerating the development of therapies for pediatric rare diseases including strategic plan: accelerating the development of therapies for pediatric rare diseases* | July 2014 |
| *Guidance for Industry, Duchenne muscular dystrophy, developing drugs for the treatment over the spectrum of disease* prepared and submitted by Parent Project Muscular Dystrophy (PPMD) to the FDA | June 25, 2014 |

Section IX.E.4) and is not specific to MD drug development; the other document is specific for MD, but is limited to DMD drug development.

There are a number of key hurdles common to the approval of all potential products to treat MD, either as a rare disease or as a form of MD, that can benefit from the advancement in DMD/BMD clinical drug development. To facilitate discussion of these hurdles, the first document, highlighting rare diseases, will be discussed, followed by a discussion of the Parent Project Muscular Dystrophy (PPMD) document, highlighting challenges that may have a wider applicability to non-DMD types of MD.

FDA's report and strategic plan on the complex issues in developing drugs and biological products for rare diseases is a useful backdrop for insights into this complex problem. The report is the result of efforts that started in 2012 when the U.S. Congress passed the FDA *Safety and Innovation Act*, which mandated holding a public meeting to encourage and accelerate the development of new therapies for pediatric rare disease as well as issuing a report that includes a strategic plan to address such therapies. The FDA held that meeting on January 6–8, 2014, for the Agency to solicit input from various stakeholders. The important issues that were discussed at the meeting included:

- The need for more comprehensive information about the natural history of most rare diseases.
- The importance of public–private, public–public (interagency and intergovernmental), and international partnerships in providing resources and facilitating data collection.
- Recommendations for greater involvement and a more active role for patients and caregivers in therapeutic product development.
- The invaluable contribution of advocacy groups in the development process to educate and recruit patients, and to assist in endpoint selection.
- The concept that patients' and families' willingness to accept risk for participation in clinical trials, and for adopting new therapies, may be greater for those affected by serious and life-threatening rare diseases.
- Methods to overcome the challenges of trial design, such as flexible drug development programs, adaptive trial designs, enrichment strategies, and master protocols.
- Endpoint development and acceptance for use in registration trials (e.g., patient reported outcomes and surrogates).
- The ways in which benefit–risk assessments guide regulatory decision making.

Several important issues were raised that fell outside of the FDA's jurisdiction, including issues dealing with reimbursement and the governance and management of patient registries. The reimbursement topic, while critically important to families with MD, is beyond the scope of this chapter. Patient registries are further discussed in Chapter 14.

Highlights of the FDA Report [1], as pertinent to MD, are provided below. Key hurdles and challenges are highlighted in *italics*.

## Clinical Trial Design Issues

According to the report, and many researchers, to effectively study drugs that can be used to treat a disease, researchers must fully understand the disease's natural history, the term used to describe how a disease would evolve if no treatment were given.

*At present, the natural history of all nine types of MD is not fully known. Given the wide variation between the various types of MD, this issue is problematic.*

The organization of natural history studies and disease registries is needed.

*At present, these studies and registries are not standardized, transparent, nor compatible regarding data collection among multiple database holders.*

*There is no consensus on how to determine endpoints for clinical trials that are clinically meaningful to patients with rare diseases.*

It was suggested at the FDA meeting that patient advocacy groups could be hubs for data collection and could help facilitate development of patient-reported outcomes for patients with specific diseases. Other sources could include published case studies, cross-sectional analyses, and prospective longitudinal natural history studies with information on phenotypic and genotypic characteristics of the disease, available biomarkers, and clinical manifestations.

*According the FDA report, **the greatest challenge in designing and interpreting clinical trials in rare diseases is the small numbers of patients available for clinical studies**.* Such small numbers of patients, if studied using conventional study design, are often unable to generate enough data to establish the efficacy and safety of the drug. Compounding this challenge is the fact that the few patients who are available for the study may exhibit varying signs of the disease or react to medications intended to treat their condition in different ways. New methods to address these challenges include various crossover designs, and use of historical control studies and enrichment strategies.

## The Benefit–Risk Assessment

It was acknowledged that patients, physicians, and regulators are willing to accept greater risks when dealing with serious diseases, and that the FDA promotes transparency in informing patients through informed consent and appropriate product labeling once the product is approved.

Risk tolerance would be expected to change as more treatments became available for a particular condition.

Parents from both the panel and the audience agreed that delaying disease progression in order to give their child a more fulfilling childhood experience would be beneficial. The uncertainty of the level of risk of an experimental intervention in order to delay disease progression was contrasted with the certainty of progressive deterioration and death due to the disease in certain forms of MD.

An important decision that is made when developing products for the treatment of rare pediatric diseases is whether there are sufficient data to support giving an experimental product to a child. This decision becomes more critical in first-in-human testing of a product for rare and life-threatening diseases with no known treatments. The panelists focused on three concepts that help to inform this decision: (1) the desired clinical benefit; (2) the probability and nature of the harms (i.e., risks) that may be acceptable to attain those benefits; and (3) the amount of uncertainty about each that is tolerable.

The panelists agreed that when considering whether the risks of an experimental product are either "reasonable" or "justified," both the type of harm that the product might cause, and likelihood that the harm may occur should be considered. *There was consensus that patients' and families' attitudes about benefit–risk should be solicited as part of the process, but it was acknowledged that these attitudes may change over time, with disease progression.* Patient advocates noted that stabilization may be seen as a reasonable benefit, as opposed to the ideal of a cure, and that even the risks for certain harms may be acceptable given the potential for slowed progression of the disease.

## Long-Term Safety Concerns

Because *clinical trials for rare disease therapies are often too small to definitively ascertain a drug's complete safety profile*, for example, failing to reveal uncommon adverse events (AEs), it is important to perform long-term safety assessments (e.g., pharmacovigilance).

## Patient Registries

A patient registry is a list or database of patient information that scientists and researchers can use to keep track of patients who have participated in clinical trials, including all relevant study information, to monitor potential long-term health effects of a given therapy and shape future clinical trials.

The report discussed the value of patient registries in moving clinical research forward. Patient registries can: (1) improve patient recruitment; (2) identify possible patient cohorts for study; (3) serve as a lead-in to natural history studies; (4) integrate patient reported and clinical data from multiple sources into a single repository; (5) stimulate new research and lead to new scientific insights; and (6) enhance creative data mining within and across disorders. When developing a new registry, the following should be taken into consideration: (1) the purpose of the registry; (2) the process of data (identified and de-identified) collection, management, and analyses across multiple platforms; (3) the data curator's role; (4) the type of informed consent needed (restricted or broad access); (5) Institutional Review Board and

Federal Information Security Management Act requirements; (6) data sources (patient, family, care-giver, and healthcare provider); (7) uses of common and unique data elements; and (8) options for data updates. *It is important to further develop partnerships and collaborations between stakeholders in the rare disease community*, and to agree upon the use of common and unique data elements in order to contribute to the sharing of data.

In the context of addressing clinical trial hurdles, patient registries are another tool used to monitor outcomes in patients after the trial is complete. Patient registries allow for long-term follow-up of patients and can foster relationships among patients with rare diseases, their caregivers, healthcare providers, and drug developers. For additional information on patient registries, see Chapter 14.

## Dose Selection

Other clinical trial challenges include determining the adequate drug exposure (what doses to study and what duration of exposure to assess) and the appropriate size for a safety database.

The report suggested, with regard to dose selection, that clinical trials should assess the safety of a range of doses, rather than focusing on a single dose. Suggestions, by panelists interviewed in the report, were made for ways to explore the safety of doses (e.g., adaptive dose finding, and use of biomarkers in dose finding and dose response).

## Gene Therapy

The spectrum of diseases for which gene transfers or therapies (hereafter referred to as gene therapies) may be used is wide-ranging. Since children potentially have many years of life ahead of them, *the issue of possible long-term permanent effects of gene therapy is critical*. These issues include the need to address long-term safety risks for children and the requirement for long-term safety follow-up. This session focused on a discussion of the development of products with uncertainty regarding their long-term benefits and risks.

Gene therapy may provide the prospect of a cure or substantial amelioration of a condition after a single administration of the product. *Patients may also incur gene-therapy-related harms, which may be prolonged or which may appear only after a long interval following treatment. For this reason, long-term follow-up is critical for gene therapy trials.* The decision to participate in trials requiring long-term safety follow-up is based on the natural history of the disease, the stage of disease, and whether long-term follow-up is prohibitive. This decision is also dependent upon whether other treatment options exist.

## Statistical Considerations

Bayesian methods combine prior information, such as that gathered in previous trials on a related product or the same product on a different population, with current trial data on an endpoint of interest (e.g., an adverse event rate), in order to form conclusions about the endpoint. Bayesian statistical methods can be used to make inferences about rare diseases in pediatric populations. *Challenging issues with studying rare diseases in pediatric populations include dealing with small sample sizes and estimation of the occurrence of rare events*. Bayesian methods can be used to overcome these issues. They provide a way to learn from evidence as it accumulates.

A full discussion of biostatistics is beyond the scope of this book; however, additional details can be found in FDA's final guidance document on Bayesian statistics titled, Guidance for the Use of Bayesian Statistics in Medical Device Clinical Trials.

## Lack of U.S. Regulatory Precedence

Common issues in drug development for rare diseases include the *small numbers of patients with the individual disease available for study*, *phenotypic heterogeneity*, *and often, a lack of regulatory precedence. The lack of regulatory precedence often means there is a lack of accepted endpoints*, *outcome assessment measures*, *instruments*, *and tools for the study of the disease*.

FDA plans to issue guidance to facilitate understanding of these common rare disease issues. Although *there is no deliverable specific to pediatrics or MD associated with this document*, some of the common issues in rare disease drug development, such as the small numbers of patients available for study, are compounded when developing drugs for children. Therefore, FDA advice on managing these common issues should be helpful to developers of therapies for pediatric rare diseases.

## Call for Additional Patient Participation

Patient participation in the process of drug development is important because they can provide the unique perspective on their disease, its effect on daily life, and the tolerability of currently available therapies. Through an understanding of the patients' and their caregivers' perspectives, developers can ensure that potential treatment effects on aspects of daily life that are important to patients are adequately captured in clinical trials. Further, this information can be helpful to FDA's review of applications for new drugs, particularly when the impact of a disease on patients is not well understood or endpoints for studying drugs for a disease are not clearly defined or established.

The *Patient-Focused Drug Development Program* provides a mechanism for obtaining patients' and caregivers input on specific disease areas, and FDA has committed to examining 20 disease areas over five years. Considerations in the selection process included disease areas:

- That are chronic, symptomatic, or affect functioning and activities of daily living
- For which aspects of the disease are not formally captured in clinical trials
- For which there are currently no therapies or very few therapies, or the available therapies do not directly affect how a patient feels or functions.

For each disease area selected, the agency is conducting a public meeting to discuss the disease and its effect on patients' daily lives, the types of treatment benefits that matter most to patients, and patients' and caregivers' perspectives on the adequacy of available therapies. These meetings include participation of FDA review divisions, the relevant patient community, and other interested stakeholders.

## PPMD Report

Additional insights into the complexities and hurdles to successfully conduct MD research can be gleaned from the PPMD-initiated FDA Guidance Document [2] on DMD/BMD, published July 2014, with key excerpts and thoughts summarized below.

## Lack of Specific MD Regulatory Guidance

The first hurdle, identified on Page 2 of the PPMD report, is that—with the exception of their own guidance (which is subject to change, may or may not be approved by the FDA, and is focused only on DMD/BMD)—the *U.S. lacks specific guidance for the clinical development of treatments for any other type of MD.*

In response to a lack of specific guidance in the U.S., the PPMD guidance discusses three regulatory pathways for expedited approval, in addition to traditional drug approval.

Please note that *these regulatory pathways are not unique to MD* and they are already established:

1. Priority review
2. Accelerated approval
3. Breakthrough or fast track

It should be noted that, like other U.S. guidance documents (and contrary to EU regulatory guidance, which does hold legal force), the *DMD guidance does not establish legally enforceable responsibilities.*

Although probably the best understood of the MDs, the natural history of DMD/BMD is not 100% understood or fully charted, despite many years of funding by government and advocacy groups, such as the Muscular Dystrophy Association (MDA). Given the *paucity of natural history understanding for some of the other types of MDs*, it has been discovered that the course of disease for DMD can be significantly altered by therapies such as long-term glucocorticoids and the management of spinal deformity. Additional details regarding regulatory guidance are provided in Chapter 10.

## The Benefit–Risk Assessment

The DMD guidance generally supports the rare disease discussion regarding the risk/benefit assessment, in that parents of the DMD population are willing to accept more uncertainty and take greater risk early on, because of the predictable and severe outcomes of the disease. Importantly, for patients with other types of MDs, the guidance recommends that the FDA better incorporate the perspective of patients and families into the benefit–risk assessment.

Unlike traditional clinical trial development, sponsors were advised to quantify the preferences of patients and family members, when feasible.

For DMD, *caregivers were willing to accept a serious risk when balanced with a non-curative treatment, even absent lifespan improvement.* In essence, stabilization of the child's progression was considered a benefit worth a serious risk; however, caregivers indicated a limit to their risk tolerance in that they would not accept a risk of death and a risk of additional lifelong disability for a drug that stopped or slowed progression.

## Delay to Diagnosis

*DMD is like other types of MD in that there can be a significant delay to diagnosis.* Despite early signs of weakness, parents may not voice their concerns or local healthcare professionals not familiar with MD may delay in pursuing testing. The delay can be substantial—as long as 2.5 years according to a MD-STARnet report and other sources [3, 4]. It has also been reported that teachers may notice clinical signs and development delays that were not recognized by health professionals. This lack of awareness suggests that the education of practitioners is critical to shortening the diagnostic odyssey (See the American Academy of Pediatrics statement on www.childmuscleweakness.org).

# Differences in Diagnostic Testing

*Not all types of MD can be diagnosed with accuracy and some subtypes of certain types of MD may not yet be identified.*

Further complicating matters is the *difficulty due to heterogeneity in multiple types of MDs.* For clinical trial participation, and in the author's experience of reviewing the literature, a molecular diagnosis is preferred over a clinical diagnosis. This helps to decrease the variation within the patient population and increase the probability of success for targeted therapies; however, even with DMD, as many as ~5% of mutations are undetectable by standard genomic analysis [5, 6].

Because our understanding of genetics is evolving, *patients who have been screened by older techniques may need to be re-tested in order to more accurately diagnosis their mutations.* Barriers to obtaining the latest genetic testing include: reluctance to visit caregiver, financial (cost), reluctance to give blood or other tissue sample, and inadequate healthcare provider education. It has been noted that because of the potential for early intervention, newborn genotypic screening is recommended, but has not yet been fully worked out. Barriers for early diagnosis include reluctance of health insurers to pay for this service due to increased cost, need for informed consent and accuracy and interpretation of the tests, meaning that genotype alone does not determine classification of all patients and cannot replace the clinical assessment.

# Natural History

As mentioned earlier, although significant advances have been made, *the natural history is not understood for all types or subtypes of the nine forms of MD.* Further work is needed to elucidate these time courses. As the PPMD paper points out, significant work was done for DMD to enhance the understanding of DMD natural history from additional data from registries and the placebo arms of industry trials. These approaches could be used for other types of MD, especially in light of the paucity of patients that can be identified and are willing to enroll in clinical trials.

# Testing and Evaluation of Clinical Endpoints with Validation

*Additional work is needed to identify clinically validated endpoints for clinical trials*; however, significant progress has been made for DMD that may apply to other types of MD. For example, Timed Function tests, such as the six-minute walk test (aka 6MWT—one of the most commonly used primary outcome measures in clinical development programs), can be used to assess progression of MD. Stair climbing, and strength tests, including manual muscle testing, quantitative lower and upper limb testing, and some patient reported outcomes, may have applicability for other types of MD in the clinical trial setting.

It should be noted that *concurrent medical management may alter the course of MD disease* and this has certainly been the case for DMD where glucocorticoids and other interventions have altered (improved) the natural course of the MD and these factors need to be accounted for in clinical trial drug development. For example, a Cochrane review concluded that for DMD, glucocorticoid corticosteroids improve muscle strength and function over six months to two years.

The loss of clinical milestones is a hallmark of disease progression in DMD, but may be true for other types of MD as well. For example, a number of ambulatory functions and milestones are listed and include:

- Unable to jump, hop, and run
- Loss of standing from the floor
- Loss of transition from lying supine to sitting
- Loss of stair climbing
- Loss of ability to stand from a chair
- Loss of ability to walk independently (defined by the inability to perform a 10 m walk/run)
- Loss of standing in place

  And non-ambulatory milestones:

- Loss of ability to reach overhead
- Loss of ability to reach the scalp
- Loss of ability to self-feed without adaptations (hand to mouth)
- Loss of ability to place hands to table top
- Loss of ability to use a computer (distal hand function)

*Although the focus of most research is on the ambulatory MD patient population, outcome measures will also need to be validated for patients in the non-ambulant population* and multiple scales are discussed in the PPMD document that may apply to other types of MD as well.

## Heterogeneity

As noted elsewhere, the goal of therapeutics in MD is to slow or stabilize disease progression in comparison to that expected from natural history. Heterogeneity among patients means that some patients with MD may experience more aggressive forms of progression than others. These subtleties need to be addressed in clinical trials and can include:

- Future progression due to disease severity, stage of disease, and known natural history
- The age at loss of clinically meaningful milestones as a surrogate for disease severity

- Imbalance of the ages of study participants
- Imbalances in gender (not discussed in the PPMD paper, but important nonetheless)
- Genetic predictors of disease progression (mutations)
- Genetic modifiers (based on genetic screening that may identify genetic polymorphisms in other genes as well)
- Previous treatments (e.g., glucocorticoids)
- Previous adaptive treatments (splinting, orthotic devices, corsets, etc.)
- Physical therapy (length, type, and progress).

## Other Obstacles

In addition to the hurdles identified in FDA's rare disease and PPMD documents, other factors have hampered MD drug development. For example, animal models of MD do not accurately reflect human disease; thus, the majority of drugs tried in animal models have failed in human clinical trials [7, 8]. As a result, increased rigor and higher standards are needed in the preclinical space. Current data suggest a tendency to move to MD clinical trials too soon and based on insufficient data [9, 10].

Other hurdles not already discussed include:

- Difficulty in defining and measuring the rate of change in slowly progressing disease conditions.
- Variety and differences in the genetic mode of transmission over the nine types of MD (e.g., autosomal dominant inheritance, autosomal recessive inheritance, germline mosaic [resulting from a mutation during development that is propagated to only a subset of the adult cells, such as sperm or eggs], de novo mutations, etc.).
- Heterogeneity of the phenotypes within each form of MD with varying treatment goals at each stage.
- Few patients being available or eligible for study in clinical trials. Although already stated, on the positive side—for example, for drug developers—it should be noted that because of the paucity of patients eligible for clinical trials, that the FDA is willing to classify MD candidates as orphan drugs. As orphans, they would garner significant advantages for the sponsor, such as regulatory exclusivity and reduced fees during the application process.
- Pediatric neuromuscular disease presents a challenge because patients lose muscle function as they grow into adolescence. Therapies, if not definitively curative, must provide a benefit–risk ratio acceptable to patients as well as caregivers; these two parties may not calculate the benefit–risk ratio in the same way.

For additional details, see Chapter 6 titled, "Transition from Childhood to Adult in Patients with Muscular Dystrophy" by Drs. Kathryn Wagner and Elba Y. Gerena Maldonado.

# Summary

A major challenge in developing therapies for DMD is that there is considerable variation in the severity and rate of disease progression in different individuals. Other hurdles include: difficulty in defining and measuring the rate of change in this slowly progressing disease; variation in the goals of treatment at each stage of DMD; and the fact that few patients are available or eligible for study in clinical trials.

Driven by the desperate need for a cure, governments and U.S. patient advocacy groups for patients with DMD (and its cousin, BMD) have led the way for patients with other types of MD, providing a surrogate pathway for other patient advocacy groups.

Europe is focusing on providing more detailed regulatory guidance, in line with its historical guidance for drug developers, but, while encouraging, this is limited. For example, in its only MD guidance, the primary focus is on male children with DMD and does not fully address parameters for women, men, and female children. The guideline also includes only a few references to BMD patients.

The U.S. is relying on current programs already in place and needed to solicit help from patient advocacy groups, such as the PPMD, in order to provide regulatory guidance. The current lack of detailed regulatory guidance adds risk to sponsors' drug development programs. Justifiably starting with DMD, the most severe form of MD, additional regulatory guidance along the lines of that provided by PPMD is desperately needed to de-risk the programs of sponsors developing treatments for the other forms of MD, such as FSHD.

Once drug developers identify enough patients to study, but before moving to clinical trials, they need to have a minimum understanding of the natural history for each type of MD and make sure that the preclinical data package justifies the risk/benefit to the patient (and caregivers).

Other hurdles to product approval for MD include the lack of protein identification and complete understanding of the mechanism of action in certain types of MD (e.g., FSHD), and lack of regulatory agreement on primary and secondary endpoints in the U.S. For example, scientific debate continues on whether Sarepta Therapeutics can use dystrophin as a surrogate endpoint for registration purposes.

Until clinical endpoints and other key clinical trial design features are provided in U.S. and EU regulatory guidance, sponsors of drugs will need to collaborate with regulatory agencies on a case-by-case basis and early solicitation is encouraged.

# References

1. Report: complex issues in developing drugs and biological products for rare diseases and accelerating the development of therapies for pediatric rare diseases including strategic 2014. http://www.fda.gov/downloads/RegulatoryInformation/Legislation/FederalFood DrugandCosmeticActFDCAct/SignificantAmendmentstotheFDCAct/FDASIA/UCM404104. pdf. Accessed 10 Dec 2014.

2. Guidance for Industry, Duchenne muscular dystrophy, developing drugs for the treatment over the spectrum of disease. 2014. http://www.parentprojectmd.org/site/DocServer/Guidance_Document_Submission_-_Duchenne_Muscular_Dystrop.pdf?docID=15283. Accessed 10 Dec 2014.
3. Ciafaloni E, Fox DJ, Pandya S, et al. Delayed diagnosis in DMD: data from the MD Surveillance, Tracking and Research Network (MD STARnet). J Pediatr. 2009;155:380–5.
4. Bushby KMD, Hill A, Steele JG. Failure of early diagnosis in symptomatic DMD. Lancet. 1999;353:557–8.
5. Khelifi MM, Ishmukhametova A, Khau Van Kien P, et al. Pure intronic rearrangements leading to aberrant pseudoexon inclusion in dystrophinopathy: a new class of mutations? Hum Mutat. 2011;32(4):467–75. doi:10.1002/humu.21471. Epub 10 Mar 2011.
6. Gurvich OL, Tuohy TM, Howard MT, et al. DMD pseudoexon mutations: splicing efficiency, phenotype, and potential therapy. Ann Neurol. 2008;63(1):81–9.
7. Landis SC, et al. A call for transparent reporting to optimize the predictive value of preclinical research. Nature. 2012;490(11):187–91.
8. Henderson VC, Kimmelman J, Fergusson D, Grimshaw JM, Hackam DG. Threats to validity in the design and conduct of preclinical efficacy studies: a systematic review of guidelines for in vivo animal experiments. PLoS Med. 2013;10(7):e1001489.
9. Mullard A. Reliability of "new drug target" claims called into question. Nat Rev. 2011; 10:643–4.
10. Prinz F, Schlange T, Asadullah K. Believe it or not: how much can we rely on published data on potential drug targets? Nat Rev Drug Discov. 2011;10:712. doi:10.1038/nrd3439-c1. http://www.nature.com/nrd/journal/v10/n9/full/nrd3439-c1.html. Accessed 9 Dec 2014.

# Chapter 12
# Pharmaceutical Products and Non-pharmaceutical Interventions as Potential Treatments for Patients with Muscular Dystrophy

Raymond A. Huml

## Treatments for Patients with Muscular Dystrophy

Despite being medically recognized for over 150 years, with hundreds of millions of dollars put to work through champion organizations such as the Muscular Dystrophy Association (MDA) and pharmaceutical sponsors, there is currently no cure for any form of muscular dystrophy (MD). However, at no time in the history of MD has the future looked brighter. With over 240 studies listed in the U.S.—and at least 11 candidates in the later phases of drug development (e.g., Phase II or Phase III)—the stage is set for positive change.

It is the author's opinion that more groundwork needs to be laid, such as the conduct of natural history studies, establishment of more global patient registries, and completion of additional genetic and molecular studies, to better understand MD and to identify promising targets. Indeed, it has historically proven difficult to find preclinical and animal models of disease. However, as these 240+ studies are completed, it is hoped that the mechanism of disease will become better elucidated, more targets will be identified, and more companies will be willing to invest in clinical trials.

It is hoped that pharmaceutical research into gene therapy or stem cell therapy will ultimately provide treatment to stop the progression of some types of MD and possibly provide a cure.

Current treatment is designed to help prevent or reduce deformities in the joints and the spine and to allow people with MD to remain mobile as long as possible. Non-pharmaceutical therapies include range-of-motion exercises, mobility aids, and assisted breathing. Other procedures can include surgery, mainly for contractures, scoliosis, and heart problems. Although current treatments are critically

R.A. Huml, M.S., D.V.M., R.A.C. (✉)
Biosimilars Center of Excellence, Quintiles Inc., Emperor Boulevard 4820,
Durham, NC 27703, USA
e-mail: raymond.huml@quintiles.com

© Springer International Publishing Switzerland 2015
R.A. Huml (ed.), *Muscular Dystrophy*, DOI 10.1007/978-3-319-17362-7_12

important for patients with MD, this chapter will be mainly limited to a discussion of pharmaceutical treatments.

For those unfamiliar with the (largely Western) milestones within the clinical trial paradigm, a brief overview is provided just below.

## Brief Overview of Clinical Trial Development

To understand the pharmaceutical product approval (aka "registration") process, it is important to be aware of the clinical trial drug development paradigm. The ultimate goal is to put the pieces of the development puzzle together as required by regulatory agencies, in order to get a drug, biologic, or device to market in the shortest time possible, with the fewest resources, and in the safest and most effective manner.

The process starts with testing many molecules in the laboratory—in vitro (using cells outside their normal biological context in a laboratory environment) and in vivo (in living organisms), proceeds to preclinical testing in animals, and then to human testing along the following paradigm:

- Discovery Phase
- Preclinical Phase
- Phase I, II, III clinical trials
- Marketing Phase
- Phase IV clinical trials.

Figure 12.1 was taken from a presentation by the FDA which describes the general plan for overall drug development. Subsequent sections of this chapter will demonstrate how governments, patient advocacy groups, and pharmaceutical companies are currently working in all phases of drug development, with the majority of work being conducted in the lower half of the foundation, but a few promising candidates pushing all the way to later phase clinical testing.

As the scientific (e.g., pathophysiology, mechanism of action [MOA], effect of intervention) and clinical data (post IND phase, such as early and later phase clinical testing) are collected and analyzed, it is sent to regulatory agencies for review and feedback on the progress of the clinical development program. After preclinical testing in the laboratory and in animals, regulatory agencies (the FDA in the U.S.) must give approval before human trials may commence.

In Phase I trials, healthy human volunteers are typically given various doses of the compound in order to study its pharmacokinetics (PK), pharmacodynamics (PD), and, to some extent, its safety. Phase II trials are generally designed to elucidate a safe and effective dosage range in a limited number of patients with the condition the drug was developed to treat. Finally, Phase III clinical trials are conducted on large numbers of patients with the condition for which the drug was developed in order to assess the drug's safety and efficacy.

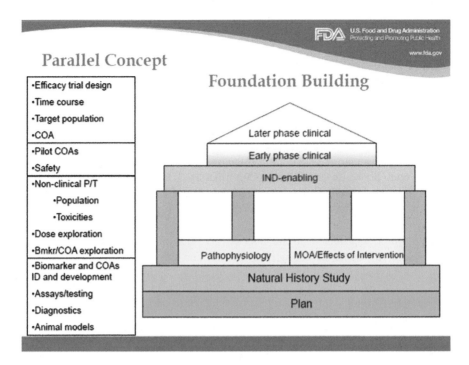

**Fig. 12.1** FDA foundation building for clinical trial drug development

Once all of the required information from the multiple trials is collected and analyzed, it is submitted for regulatory approval in the form of written reports. A team of experts from multiple disciplines reviews portions of the data package and determines whether the drug is both safe and effective for the indication for which it was developed. Of interest is the fact that the FDA simply approves the proposed labeling (package insert) for the drug, and not the drug itself, yet it is illegal to market a drug for treatment of any disease without FDA-approved labeling. After the labeling is approved, the product continues to be monitored in an ever-enlarging population of patients as long as it remains on the market. After a drug is in general use, its sponsor may compare it with others used for the same indication either to bolster superiority claims or to study further the safety and efficacy of the product as part of a regulatory commitment at the time of original FDA approval. Such activities are known as Phase IV post-marketing studies.

Although this is the general paradigm for the approval of many drugs, certain exceptions can be made, because of issues such as the ethical conundrum of giving a placebo in lieu of a potential disease modifying treatment to a patient afflicted with MD. In these cases, some groups, such as PMDD, advocate for a comparison between the active drug and the expected natural history course of the disease. Although this is entirely understandable, given the variation with MD—even within families—this may prove difficult unless additional natural history studies are conducted.

## *Approved Products and Treatments*

There is only one product tentatively approved for the treatment of MD anywhere in the world. As mentioned earlier, PTC Therapeutics' ataluren was granted marketing authorization (tentative approval) in the EU under the trade name Translarna™ for the treatment of DMD in ambulatory patients aged five years and older. Translarna™ is approved to treat the underlying cause of DMD. The European Medicines Agency has designated ataluren as an orphan medicinal product and the FDA has granted orphan drug designation to ataluren for the treatment of DMD.

The ongoing Phase III Ataluren Confirmatory Trial is a randomized, double-blind, placebo-controlled trial designed to confirm the safety and efficacy results seen in an earlier Phase IIb study. The confirmatory study was designed to enroll 220 participants at approximately 58 sites in North America, South America, Europe, Israel, Asia, and Australia. Successful results of this trial would provide the basis for a full approval decision in the EU and the U.S., as well as in other countries.

According to DuchenneConnect: [1]

> Based on estimates regarding patient enrollment, initial, top-line data from the Phase III clinical trial were expected in mid-2015. If trial results support approval and FDA approves their application, Translarna™ could be available in the U.S. as early as the second half of 2016. PTC plans to apply for approval in other countries following U.S. approval.

## *Potential Treatments for MD*

A total of 247 MD studies were identified (on October 30, 2014) using the search term "muscular dystrophy" on the Website titled *clinicaltrials.gov*—a government mandated Website dedicated to posting all clinical trials being conducted in the U.S. It is important to note that other studies may be ongoing—and not recognized on this Website—as they may be conducted in Europe or other non-U.S. regions. Clinical trials conducted in EU and European Economic Area (EEA) can be found at www.clinicaltrialsregister.eu.

It should be emphasized that U.S., Europe, and Japan are the only countries currently following International Conference of Harmonization (ICH) guidelines on good clinical practice and the conduct of clinical trials. This is important to note because a clinical dossier for registration purposes can be filed simultaneously in all ICH countries, though, in the author's opinion, there are still subtle differences between these geographies meaning that this is not always achievable.

It is also important to note, for those considering participating in a clinical trial outside of ICH countries, that the other countries may not have as rigorous clinical trial requirements and this should be factored into any clinical risk/benefit analysis.

**Table 12.1**   U.S. clinical trials[a] for the treatment of the nine major types of MD[b]

| Type of MD/search term | Number of clinical trials |
| --- | --- |
| Duchenne muscular dystrophy | 105 |
| Becker muscular dystrophy | 124 |
| Facioscapulohumeral muscular dystrophy | 21 |
| Congenital muscular dystrophy | 26 |
| Distal muscular dystrophy | 9 |
| Emery-Dreifuss muscular dystrophy | None[c] |
| Limb Girdle muscular dystrophy | 19 |
| Myotonic muscular dystrophy | 20 |
| Oculopharyngeal muscular dystrophy | None [1] |

[a]It should be noted that these U.S. studies do not just reflect potential pharmaceutical intervention, but also non-pharmaceutical interventions such as electrostimulation; high intensity training; antioxidants; stem cells; registries; protein supplementation; older, approved products that have not yet been studied for the treatment of MD (e.g., albuterol, oxandrolone); and diagnostic procedures (e.g., MRI)

[b]Does not include Collagen VI MD and Ullrich Congenital MD

[c]A lack of listings on clinicaltrials.gov does not mean that no clinical drug development is being conducted because some sponsors choose to conduct clinical trials outside of the U.S. See Table 12.2 where a Phase III (late stage) candidate for oculopharyngeal MD is identified

Of these 247 studies, 105 studies were found for "Duchenne muscular dystrophy" and 124 studies were found for "Becker muscular dystrophy," though it should be noted that most of these studies overlap (because they have a similar pathology), thus are double-counted and not unique. Most DMD and BMD studies focus on treatment of the heart and lungs, where complications can cause early mortality in DMD patients.

Only seven studies were found using the search term "FSH or FSHD"; however, 21 studies were discovered for FSHD using the full search term, "facioscapulohumeral muscular dystrophy," which reinforces that how one conducts a query may influence the number of studies discovered.

The rest of the studies—about half—are associated with other types of MD as depicted in Table 12.1.

## Congenital Muscular Dystrophy

Of the 26 Congenital MD studies cited, most are focused on gathering information to better understand the disease. For example, several trials are listed as natural history or genetic studies and some highlight patient- and family-reported medical information. Most of the other studies included diagnostic tests or physical therapy-type studies (e.g., lung stretch therapy).

## Distal Muscular Dystrophy

Distal muscular dystrophy was similar to Congenital MD, except with fewer studies; five out of nine studies were listed as "completed" and only two studies reported as recruiting patients.

## Limb Girdle Muscular Dystrophy

Limb Girdle muscular dystrophy was similar to Congenital and Distal MDs—meaning that most studies are focused on gathering information to better understand the disease—except that there are more molecular and genetic studies, including gene transfer and stem cell therapy, though the stem cell therapy was for patients with FSHD, not Limb Girdle MD (as accessed on November 7, 2014).

## Myotonic Muscular Dystrophy

Most myotonic muscular dystrophy studies focus on the heart and lungs with two notable exceptions: Iplex from Somaokine and Mexiletine.

According to the ADIS database, Iplex, an insulin-like growth factor, was being studied for multiple indications in the Phase II stage of drug development in Europe; however, clinical development had been suspended or discontinued for multiple indications, including MD.

Mexiletine, an orally active local anesthetic agent structurally related to lidocaine, is an approved drug (sponsor Boehringer Ingelheim). This was studied in Italy in a small number of patients with generalized dystonia, but there has been no further development since 2009, according to the ADIS database (as of November 8, 2014).

## *Duchenne Muscular Dystrophy: Mechanism of Action*

DMD and BMD account for the largest number of clinical trials and have the same MOA, being caused by a defect in the gene for the muscle protein, dystrophin. This may be inherited or may occur without a known family history of the condition [1].

Looking ahead, there is cause for optimism that the approaches being investigated in clinical trials may address the huge unmet medical need for new treatments for DMD and potentially other MDs—ideally by slowing down or halting disease progression, or providing an urgently needed cure.

Most of the clinical studies in the U.S. for DMD involve diagnostic tests to study heart and lung function, stem cell therapies, older, approved products being studied for the treatment of DMD (metformin, carvedilol, prednisone), and protein supplementation (e.g., L-arginine, creatinine, and glutamine).

Current treatments for DMD are aimed at, reducing symptoms and improving quality of life. For example, corticosteroids can help slow down the loss of muscle strength [2]. However, researchers have made great advances in their knowledge of DMD and continue to search for a cure. Several promising approaches to DMD are in the pipeline, according to the MDA [3]:

*"Exon skipping" drug candidates*, which target the mutation that occurs in the gene for dystrophin in individuals with DMD. Also known as molecular patches or antisense oligonucleotides, these are designed to skip the faulty section of this gene so that the muscle protein can be produced, hopefully reducing the symptoms of DMD. Two such products are currently in development: Sarepta's RNA-based clinical candidate, eteplirsen, and Prosensa's drisapersen [4, 5].

*Gene therapy*, aimed at introducing a healthy synthetic copy of the dystrophin gene into the muscles to restore production of dystrophin. Challenges include the fact that the dystrophin gene is too big to fit within the virus used to deliver it to muscles; and the body may respond to the virus or dystrophin with an immune reaction. Gene therapy holds great potential if these challenges can be successfully tackled.

*Reading through stop signals* by targeting a specific type of mistake in the genetic code called a nonsense mutation, which prevents the production of full-length functional proteins and affects 10–15% of boys with DMD. For example, PTC Therapeutics' drug candidate, Ataluren (PTC124) [6], has potential to enable the cell to read through premature nonsense stop signals and make dystrophin.

*Stem cell therapy*, where donor cells are injected with the aim of creating healthy muscle fibers. It may also be possible to isolate the patient's own stem cells, grow them in the laboratory, correct the genetic defect with gene therapy, and transplant them back into the patient.

*Utrophin upregulation*, aimed at increasing levels of utrophin, a protein that is functionally similar to dystrophin. Summit's investigational oral small molecule SMT C1100 is in early clinical trials for this use [7].

*Reducing muscle damage* is another goal of ongoing research. For example, Dart Therapeutics' HT-100 is an orally available, small molecule drug candidate intended to reduce accumulation of scar tissue and inflammation, and to promote healthy muscle fiber regeneration [8].

**Selected Case Examples**

Hundreds of pharmaceutical candidates, interventions, and studies are posted on *clinicaltrials.gov*, and, according to a Web search on December 5, 2014, a total of 111 candidates and therapies for the treatment of MD (including protein supplements and drugs previously approved for indications other than MD) have advanced to the Phase II ($n = 72$) or Phase III ($n = 39$) stage of clinical drug development. These pharmaceutical candidates represent a significant investment in capital, as well as caregiver and patient time, effort and, in some cases, biological samples.

For Phase II candidates, many trials are studying older, approved drugs and supplements, but in new ways or for new indications (e.g., prednisone, coenzyme Q, metformin, creatine, glutamine), but some candidates appear to be novel, such as GSK's GSK2402968, idebenone, drisapersen, and eteplirsen, to name a few.

For Phase III candidates, with few exceptions, studies mainly focus on the treatment of DMD/BMD. For example, some Phase III studies are being conducted in patients with Miyoshi myopathy ($n = 1$), myotonic dystrophy ($n = 2$), or rare diseases like Bethlem myopathy and Ullrich Congenital MD ($n = 1$ [same trial to study potential treatment for both diseases]).

Selected novel therapies, in both Phase II and Phase III phases of drug development, are summarized in Table 12.2 below.

Case examples for some of these candidates are provided at the end of this chapter.

**Table 12.2** Selected candidates in the late stage MD pipeline

| Primary drug name | Mechanism of action | Phase of drug development | MD target[a] |
|---|---|---|---|
| Tadalafil | Phosphodiesterase 5 inhibitor | Phase III | DMD |
| **Ataluren** | **Dystrophin stimulant** | **Phase III in U.S.; tentatively approved in the EU** | **DMD, BMD** |
| Idebenone | Reducing agent, apoptosis inhibitor | Phase III | DMD |
| **Drisapersen** | **Dystrophin stimulant** | **Pre-registration** | **DMD** |
| **Eteplirsen** | **Dystrophin stimulant** | **Phase III** | **DMD** |
| Trehalose dihydrate | Protein aggregate inhibitor | Phase III | Oculopharyngeal MD |
| Intramuscular transplant of muscle-derived stem cells & adipose mesenchymal cells | Stimulation and creation of new (normal) muscle cells | Phase III | FSHD |
| PRO-053, PRO-045, PRO-044 | Dystrophin stimulants | Phase II | DMD |
| Pemirolast® | Histamine release inhibitor, reduction of vascular inflammation | Phase II | DMD, BMD |
| Halofuginone hydrobromide | Angiogenesis inhibitor, collagen Type I inhibitor | Phase II | DMD |

(continued)

**Table 12.2** (continued)

| Primary drug name | Mechanism of action | Phase of drug development | MD target[a] |
|---|---|---|---|
| Givinostat | TNF alpha antagonist, IL 1b antagonist, histone deacetylase inhibitor, IL6 receptor antagonist | Phase II | DMD |
| Follistatin | Human growth and differentiation factor 8 antagonist | Phase II | BMD |
| **ATYR-1940** | **Histidine-tRNA ligase modulator** | **Phase II** | **FSHD** |

Compounds highlighted in bold are discussed in greater detail as case studies later in this chapter
[a]Some of these candidates for the treatment of MD are being studied for the treatment of other diseases. In these cases, only the MD target is identified

## Case Example: Ataluren [9]

PTC Therapeutics is developing ataluren (Translarna™) for the treatment of multiple genetic disorders including cystic fibrosis and DMD. Ataluren is formulated as a powder for suspension in water or milk. It is an orally administered, small-molecule compound that targets nonsense mutations. Nonsense mutations are single-point alterations in DNA that introduce a premature translation termination codon, when transcribed into mRNA. This change halts the ribosomal translation process at an earlier site than normal, producing a truncated, non-functional protein. Ataluren allows the cellular machinery to read through premature stop codons in mRNA, and thereby enables the translation process to produce full-length, functional proteins. Specifically, ataluren is designed to mediate the cystic fibrosis transmembrane conductance regulator (CFTR) chloride channel for cystic fibrosis and the functional production of dystrophin for DMD. Ataluren is conditionally approved for the treatment of nonsense-mutation DMD (or nmDMD) in the EU, Norway, Iceland, and Lichtenstein.

PTC is conducting a multinational Phase III clinical trial (Ataluren Confirmatory Trial in DMD, or ACT DMD) in support of the conditional approval of ataluren for nonsense mutation DMD. In December 2014, PTC announced that it had commenced a rolling submission of a New Drug Application (NDA) to the FDA for Translarna™ for the treatment of nmDMD. Phase III development in cystic fibrosis is underway in the U.S., Canada, and the EU. Phase II trials were planned for other diseases; however, development for these indications has been suspended to focus on DMD and cystic fibrosis.

According to PTC Therapeutics, ataluren is the first product in the world approved to treat nonsense mutations that cause DMD. Aminoglycosides have also demonstrated an ability to selectively promote read-through of nonsense mutations;

however, these agents require parenteral administration and the high doses involved increase the risk of serious toxicity. PTC aims to overcome these limitations by developing an orally administered non-aminoglycoside.

## Case Example: Drisapersen [10, 11]

According to ADIS, Prosensa Holding N.V. (aka Prosensa) is developing drisapersen, a 2′-O-methyl antisense oligonucleotide, for the treatment of DMD. DMD is caused by deletion or duplication of exons, or point mutations, in the gene that encodes dystrophin. Because of their capacity to skip an exon by blocking its inclusion during splicing, antisense oligonucleotides have the potential to correct the reading frame of DMD transcripts to yield an internally truncated dystrophin protein. Studies in cultured cells from patients with DMD have demonstrated that drisapersen efficiently induces specific skipping of exon 51. Based on the frequency of mutations in patients with DMD, drisapersen may have the ability to correct the reading frame in up to 25% of deletions, including exon 50, exon 52, exons 45–50, exons 48–50, and exons 49–50. Phase III development of a subcutaneous formulation is underway worldwide for the treatment of DMD.

In the U.S., on October 10, 2014, Prosensa announced that it had initiated the process of submission of a New Drug Application to the FDA. Drisapersen has Breakthrough Therapy Designation and Fast Track Status in the U.S., which made it eligible for a rolling review of the NDA. The submission is expected to be completed before 2015. The company announced on November 24, 2014, that it had been acquired by BioMarin Pharmaceutical Inc. Currently, Prosensa has six DMD candidates in its pipeline, drisapersen being the most advanced one. Notably, all these candidates have orphan drug status in the U.S. and the EU.

Prosensa completed a randomized, double-blind, placebo-controlled Phase III study (results announced in September 2013) on drisapersen for DMD. However, the candidate failed to meet the primary endpoint. The company started re-dosing patients in September 2014.

Prosensa has said that it intends to submit a marketing authorization application in the near future to the European Medicines Agency for conditional approval of drisapersen.

## Case Example: Eteplirsen [12]

Sarepta Therapeutics (formerly AVI BioPharma) is developing eteplirsen for the treatment of DMD—where internal exon mutations lead to the formation of truncated dystrophin proteins lacking one of the functional ends. Eteplirsen allows exon 51 to be skipped, providing altered messenger RNA (mRNA), which in turn produces a shortened but functional version of dystrophin. Eteplirsen uses Sarepta's phosphorodiamidate morpholino oligomer (PMO)-based chemistry and proprietary exon-skipping technology. Oligonucleotides based on this splicing technology do not degrade target RNA and do not lead to down-regulation of the target gene. Previously, AVI BioPharma completed a Phase I/II trial in the UK evaluating intravenously administered eteplirsen in patients with DMD. Phase III development of intravenously infused eteplirsen is underway in the U.S. Sarepta is planning to file for approval with the FDA in the near future, based on the Pre-NDA meeting.

Positive results from a phase I/II trial of intramuscularly administered eteplirsen were reported. However, the company appears to be focusing on the development of eteplirsen for intravenous administration.

A similar approach is being utilized by Sarepta to develop AVI-5038, a therapeutic candidate for DMD with the ability to skip dystrophin exon 50.

## *Case Example: ATYR-1940 [13, 14]*

aTyr Pharma is developing a protein, Resolaris™ (ATYR1940), based on naturally occurring truncated amino acyl-tRNA synthetases, called physiocrines, for the treatment of MDs, including FSHD. Phase I/II development is underway in France and the Netherlands.

Although still early in clinical development, it is interesting to note that in August 2014, aTyr Pharma initiated a Phase I/II trial evaluating the safety and tolerability of ATYR 1940 in patients with molecularly defined genetic facioscapulohumeral muscular dystrophy (ATYR1940-C-002; EudraCT2014-001753-17; NCT02239224). The randomized, double-blind, multiple ascending dose trial is intended to enroll 44 patients in France and the Netherlands. In February 2015, the company announced that the European Commission had granted orphan drug designation to Resolaris™ for the treatment of FSHD.

## References

1. Duchenne connect FAQ: Ataluran (Translarna™)—an investigational new drug for nonsense mutations by PTC therapuetics. https://www.duchenneconnect.org/en/clinical-trials/study-faq-sheets/646-ataluren-a-novel-drug-for-nonsense-mutations-by-ptc-therapeutics-inc.html. Accessed 10 Dec 2014.
2. http://www.nlm.nih.gov/medlineplus/ency/article/000705.htm. Accessed 10 Dec 2014.
3. http://www.mda.org.au/Disorders/Dystrophies/DMD-BMD.asp. Accessed 10 Dec 2014.
4. http://investorrelations.sareptatherapeutics.com/phoenix.zhtml?c=64231&p=RssLanding&cat=news&id=1904192. Accessed 10 Dec 2014.
5. http://www.reuters.com/article/2014/01/16/us-prosensa-muscledisorderdrug-idUSBREA0F1IR20140116. Accessed 10 Dec 2014.
6. http://www.prosensa.eu/technology-and-products/pipeline/drisapersen-pro051. Accessed 10 Dec 2014.
7. http://www.ptcbio.com/ataluren. Accessed 10 Dec 2014.

8. http://www.summitplc.com/programmes/duchenne-muscular-dystrophy/. Accessed 10 Dec 2014.
9. ADIS database, Ataluren. http://bi.adisinsight.com/frames.aspx. Accessed 8 Nov 2014.
10. ADIS literature search, Drisapersen. http://bi.adisinsight.com/frames.aspx. Accessed 8 Nov 2014.
11. Diseases and conditions: muscular dystrophy, treatments and drugs. Mayo Clinic. http://www.mayoclinic.org/diseases-conditions/muscular-dystrophy/basics/treatment/con-20021240. Accessed 24 Oct 2014.
12. ADIS database, Eteplirsen. http://bi.adisinsight.com/frames.aspx. Accessed 8 Nov 2014.
13. ADIS Database, ATYR-1940. http://bi.adisinsight.com/frames.aspx. Accessed 8 Nov 2014.
14. A placebo-controlled, randomized, multiple ascending dose study to evaluate the safety, tolerability, pharmacokinetics, and biological activity of ATYR1940 in adult patients with molecularly defined genetic muscular dystrophies. http://clinicaltrials.gov/show/NCT02239224. Accessed 8 Nov 2014.

# Chapter 13
# U.S. Patient Advocacy Groups

Meredith L. Huml

For newly diagnosed muscular dystrophy (MD) patients and their caregivers in the U.S., the first point of call for information and support should be the Muscular Dystrophy Association (MDA, www.mda.org). In addition, there are disease-specific groups for several of the nine forms of MD, as shown in Table 13.1.

## All Forms of MD

The MDA is the world's leading nonprofit health agency dedicated to finding treatments and cures for MD, amyotrophic lateral sclerosis (ALS), and other neuromuscular diseases. The Association does this by funding worldwide research; by providing comprehensive healthcare services and support to MDA families nationwide; and by rallying communities to fight back through advocacy, fundraising, and local engagement.

The organization is funded by individual private contributions and cooperating organizations, providing research, services, and education. Currently, over 250 research projects are funded through the MDA. Although a national group, the MDA makes its resources and information accessible through local chapters, with 200 clinics throughout the states and 100 local offices. Some 44 of those clinics are MDA/ALS centers. MDA holds annual biannual clinical and scientific conferences where cutting-edge research and clinical trial information is presented. In addition, around 3,800 children attend MDA summer camp every year, and MDA's online Transitions Center is a clearinghouse for resources to support young adults seeking employment, education, independent living, and community involvement; blogs are posted twice weekly from young adults sharing their experiences living with neuromuscular disease.

M.L. Huml (✉)
℅ Raymond A. Huml, Quintiles Inc., 4820 Emperor Blvd, Durham, NC 27703, USA

© Springer International Publishing Switzerland 2015
R.A. Huml (ed.), *Muscular Dystrophy*, DOI 10.1007/978-3-319-17362-7_13

**Table 13.1** Patient advocacy groups for MD

| Type of MD | Sources of information and support |
|---|---|
| Duchenne MD | MDA (MDA, mda.org) |
| | Parent Project Muscular Dystrophy (PPMD, http://www.parentprojectmd.org) |
| | The Foundation to Eradicate Duchenne (http://duchennemd.org) |
| | Duchenne Alliance (http://www.duchennealliance.org) |
| | Other organizations around the world are listed at http://www.parentprojectmd.org/site/PageServer?pagename=Connect_partners, http://www.treat-nmd.eu/dmd/patient-organizations/, https://www.duchenneconnect.org, & http://www.cureduchenne.org |
| Becker MD | MDA (http://mda.org/disease/becker-muscular-dystrophy) |
| Congenital MD | MDA (MDA, mda.org) |
| | Cure CMD (http://curecmd.org) |
| Distal MD | MDA (http://mda.org/disease/distal-muscular-dystrophy/types) |
| Emery-Dreifuss MD | MDA (http://www.mda.org/disease/emery-dreifuss-muscular-dystrophymda.org) |
| | National Organization for Rare Disorders (NORD, https://www.rarediseases.org) |
| Facioscapulohumeral MD (FSHD) | FSH Society (http://www.fshsociety.org) |
| | MDA (MDA, mda.org) |
| | PNW Friends of FSH Research (http://www.fshfriends.org) |
| Limb-girdle MD | MDA (MDA, mda.org) |
| | Jain Foundation (http://www.jain-foundation.org) |
| Myotonic dystrophy (DM) | MDA (MDA, mda.org) |
| | Myotonic Dystrophy Foundation (http://www.myotonic.org) |
| Oculopharyngeal MD (OPMD) | MDA (http://mda.org/disease/oculopharyngeal-muscular-dystrophy) |
| | NORD (https://www.rarediseases.org/rare-disease-information/rare-diseases/byID/1182/viewAbstract) |

MDA also hosts 150 support groups across the country. MDA's advocacy program, based in Washington, DC, seeks to make the MD community's voice heard and to expand resources for those with neuromuscular disease. By informing and educating legislators, MDA aims to accelerate development of new therapies. Individuals can sign up to be an MDA advocate and receive regular advocacy updates on the organization's web site.

The MDA publishes a quarterly magazine, *Quest Magazine*, which is sent free of charge to families registered with MDA and is also archived online at http://quest.mda.org. The organization also has an online-only *MDA/ALS Newsmagazine* at http://alsn.mda.org. MDA is also active through social media channels, including Facebook and Twitter, enabling patients and caregivers to connect with one another and providing the latest research updates.

## *Duchenne MD*

Parent Project Muscular Dystrophy (PPMD) focuses on finding an end to Duchenne MD specifically. In total, this group has invested over $45 million dollars in research, which has leveraged over $500 million in additional funding. PPMD has been involved in several steps forward for the MD community, including providing the FDA with the first-ever patient-initiated guidance to help accelerate development and review of potential therapies for Duchenne MD. PPMD also recently announced that a gene therapy study that it had funded might improve walking ability in MD. Historically, the group was instrumental in the passing of the MD Care Act in 2001. There are also a number of projects listed on their web site that need funding and lists of projects they have supported financially.

The PPMD web site has a helpful section, labeled as "Connect," which provides links for the group's monthly e-newsletter, updates on upcoming events, current research, and other MD groups. The organization has a mobile application for iPhone and Android users that informs patients of new clinical trials and other news, as well as location and contact information for nearby clinics. The PPMD Facebook and Twitter pages are regularly updated with pictures and news from the MD community, both scientific and patient-related. PPMD has also created a community page where visitors can post a profile in order to meet other members, read blogs, and share pictures. Many people who are affected by MD find that attending an event, having a chance to meet other patients or family members facing similar challenges can bring a sense of comfort and connectedness. The PPMD holds annual Connect Conferences and Meetings, typically attended by around 500 families.

There are other organizations keeping the end to Duchenne as a priority. CureDuchenne states on its website that it is a "national nonprofit that raises awareness and funds to find a cure for Duchenne muscular dystrophy." This organization has helped fund two companies (Prosensa and Sarepta) that are seeking FDA approval for drugs for MD. CureDuchenne's research investments have leveraged around $100 million from government agencies and pharmaceutical companies. In 2014, they hosted the sixth Climb for Duchenne, where "teams of people across the country can climb various mountains, hills, or tall buildings" to raise awareness and funds for CureDuchenne. The site encourages advocacy for fighting Duchenne by creating links for starting individual fundraisers.

The Foundation to Eradicate Duchenne (FED) was created in 2002 by Dana and Joel Wood, residing in Virginia, after their son was diagnosed with the disease. The Foundation's web site says it has worked with others to achieve millions of dollars in federal earmarks for Duchenne MD research and a significant increase in the attention devoted to DMD at the National Institutes of Health. Additionally, through the FED and other fundraising efforts, the group has raised nearly $10 million in private donations and worked with Congress to secure nearly $40 million in federal appropriations. While not updated frequently, this group's social network pages include several links for contact information from staff and for general questions, advocacy, and donations.

The Duchenne Alliance is an "alliance of independent non-profit organizations," with various academic and industry research projects inviting donations. The group also has plentiful blog entries and is active on Facebook and Twitter.

While the majority of patient advocacy resources focus on Duchenne, there are also resources for other types.

## Becker MD

Due to its mechanistic similarity to Duchenne MD, Becker MD is covered by many of the same groups that focus on Duchenne, particularly the MDA.

## Congenital MD

Cure CMD provides extensive resources for patients with congenital MD. The group has a mission to bring research, treatments, and in the future, a cure for CMD, by working globally together with dedicated parent, government, and research advocates. By focusing on this mission, Cure CMD aims to find and fund high potential research and clinical trials. MDA also provides extensive clinical and research funding, and other support services to individuals with CMD.

## Distal MD

The MDA supports patients with this type of MD.

## Emery-Dreifuss MD

This type of MD is also supported by the MDA, and by the National Organization for Rare Disorders, which provides links to various other resources at http://www.rarediseases.org/rare-disease-information/rare-diseases/byID/590/viewAbstract.

## Facioscapulohumeral MD

The FSH Society (Facioscapulohumeral Society) is a world leader in combating FSHD. The Society's purpose is to conduct research, increase awareness, understanding, and education on FSHD. This is especially important as FSHD may be one of the most common adult MDs, affecting men, women, and children worldwide.

MDA has also spent millions on FSH research and support services for families, and the majority of individuals are seen in MDA clinics.

The FSH Society has provided seed funds and grants to pioneering FSHD research areas and education worldwide and created an international collaborative network of patients and researchers to support research relevant to understanding the molecular genetics and causes of FSHD. The FSH Society provides strategy for FSHD research, therapeutics, and clinical trials readiness, recruiting qualified researchers and clinician-researchers, selecting research proposals, evaluating research proposals, granting fellowships, and monitoring ongoing projects and research opportunities. Grant making to FSHD researchers and clinicians is one of the largest components of the FSH Society and these efforts have led to more than 300 publications acknowledging this support in scientific journals.

Recent advances in understanding the molecular genetics and cellular biology of FSHD have led to the identification of potential therapeutic targets. The Society's main focus is to gather more support for research from the U.S. government by submitting both oral and written testimonies to Congress, all of which can be read through links on the site.

Meetings, symposia, workshops, and networking activities are one of the most successful programmatic components of the FSH Society. Through the FSH Society staff and its web site portal at www.fshsociety.org, Facebook page, Twitter account, Yahoo! Groups bulletin board, e-mail ListServ, and quarterly newsletter the *FSH Watch*, FSHD patients have found ways to be useful to one another and to basic and clinical researchers working on their disease. This group's web site is extremely abundant with information, much appreciated by the author, who is an FSHD patient herself. The support patients receive from one another through sharing their common experience is invaluable and immeasurable. The FSH Society acts as a clearinghouse for information on the FSHD disorder and on potential drugs and devices designed to alleviate the effects of the disease. It fosters communication among FSHD patients, their families and caregivers, charitable organizations, government agencies, industry, scientific researchers, and academic institutions.

The FSH Society also provides dedicated support, education, and outreach services to patients, professionals, researchers, and families in need of assistance. The Society responds to inquiries by phone, web, and e-mail from newly diagnosed patients, patients, family members and spouses of FSHD patients, and professionals.

The FSH Society helped educate and recruit patients into research studies to help facilitate the production of the world's largest resource for FSHD biomaterials that are being made available to researchers worldwide. The Society hopes that this strategy will help with better reproduction, validation, and corroboration of research results by providing the community with a high quality and high number of well-controlled FSHD cell lines that multiple research groups can independently access. Publications, literature, education, patient support, social networking, and research networking combined are the most significant components of the FSH Society.

## *Limb-Girdle MD*

There are many foundations that focus on individual subtypes of limb girdle muscular dystrophies (LGMDs), both in the U.S. and abroad. These foundations are often started by families of individuals with the disease and usually focus both on patient advocacy and on supporting research towards finding treatments and cures. MDA has also invested a lot of funding for research and support for families with LGMD.

Although LGMDs share common symptoms, the diseases are caused by mutations in a large number of genes. This large genetic diversity, the high cost of genetic analysis, and the refusal of some health insurance companies to cover genetic diagnosis make it difficult for individuals to obtain a definitive diagnosis. To address this problem, a consortium of LGMD family foundations was formed in 2014 and includes the Cecil B Day Family, Inc (LGMD2B), Coalition to Cure Calpain 3 (LGMD2A), Jain Foundation (LGMD2B), Kurt+Peter Foundation (LGMD2C), LGMD2D Foundation, LGMD2I Fund, and McColl-Lockwood Laboratory (LGMD2I).

Led by the Jain Foundation, the LGMD consortium created a new diagnostic program (http://lgmd-diagnosis.org) that offers free genetic sequencing to individuals with unexplained muscle weakness. Patients can apply for the program by taking a short quiz or their physicians can apply on their behalf using the Jain Foundation's Automated LGMD Diagnostic Assistant (ALDA—http://www.jain-foundation.org/alda) to determine eligibility. Qualified patients send in a saliva sample and receive a genetic report that includes results from a gene panel of 35 genes known to be involved in various forms of LGMD as well as other muscle diseases with similar symptoms. The diagnosis program launched in late 2014 and is already succeeding in its goal of identifying a large number of individuals with LGMDs.

Many of the LGMD consortium members focus on patient advocacy and have patient registries including the Jain Foundation, Coalition to Cure Calpain 3, LGMD2D Foundation LGMD2I Fund, and the Kurt+Peter Foundation. The identification of a large number of patients with the LGMDs studied by the foundations will help each foundation in their goals of curing each disease.

The Jain Foundation (http://jain-foundation.org) has a mission of curing muscular dystrophies caused by mutations in the dysferlin gene, which includes the clinical presentations Limb-Girdle MD type 2B (LGMD2B) and Miyoshi muscular dystrophy 1 (MMD1). The foundation is privately funded and does not solicit funding from patients or other sources. Its strategy includes funding and actively monitoring the progress of scientific research projects in key pathways towards a cure, providing financial and logistical support to promising drug candidates to accelerate them to clinical trials, funding clinical trials and studies, encouraging collaboration among scientists, and educating LGMD2B/Miyoshi patients about their disease and helping them with their diagnosis.

Coalition to Cure Calpain 3 (C3) (http://www.curecalpain3.org) was founded in 2010 for the specific purpose of funding research efforts focused on understanding the biology of and finding a cure for LGMD2A. This disease is also sometimes referred to as calpainopathy because it is caused by mutations in the calpain 3 gene. The organization was created by people with LGMD2A for people with LGMD2A, as both founders have the disease. The main focus of C3 is on supporting researchers and encouraging collaboration among scientists rather than on providing services to those who have the disease.

The LGMD2D Foundation (http://lgmd2d.org) is a non-profit private foundation whose mission is to expedite the development of a cure or therapy for Limb Girdle Muscular Dystrophy 2D (LGMD2D), which is caused by mutations in the alpha sarcoglycan protein. In addition to educating patients and physicians, the LGMD2D Foundation maintains a patient registry, funds and monitors research and progress, provides financial support to accelerate clinical trials, and encourages scientific collaboration.

The LGMD2I Research Fund (http://www.lgmd2ifund.org) is a not-for-profit focused on expediting the development of a treatment or cure for Limb Girdle Muscular Dystrophy 2I (LGMD2I), which is caused by mutations in the fukutin-related protein. The foundation does this by building a comprehensive view of the entire LGMD2I research landscape, supporting the most promising research projects, and coordinating and managing the scientific process.

The Kurt+Peter Foundation (http://kurtpeterfoundation.org) was formed by the family and friends of Kurt and Peter Frewing to raise money and direct it into the hands of the researchers who have the best shot at developing a treatment or cure for LGMD2C, which is caused by mutations in the gamma sarcoglycan gene. Since 2010, the Kurt+Peter Foundation has raised more than $1 million for research into LGMD2C. Among other initiatives, the foundation is currently funding development of an exon skipping compound that the foundation hopes will treat the majority of LGMD2C mutations.

## *Myotonic Dystrophy (DM)*

The Myotonic Dystrophy Foundation is focused on supporting and driving the research, resources, and community capacity needed to achieve the first clinical trials for myotonic dystrophy treatments, while providing comprehensive support and education to families living with this disease. The foundation's web site provides listings for support groups, a blog, details of ongoing research, and links to social media sites such as Facebook and Twitter. Both are updated regularly, and the organization is partnered with MDA. Individuals may join the Myotonic Dystrophy Family Registry, which gives the members access to research data and anonymous information regarding individuals also living with this particular genre of dystrophy.

MDA also has a focus on DM.

## *Oculopharyngeal MD (OPMD)*

This form of MD is covered by the MDA and NORD.

Outside of the patient advocacy groups, other sources of information on MD include medical, healthcare system, academic, and government institute web sites. Examples include WebMD, Medline Plus, Medscape, Genetics Home Reference, the Mayo Clinic, Johns Hopkins Medicine, the University of Maryland Medical Center, National Center for Biotechnology Information, and National Human Genome Research Institute.

Overall, patient advocacy is extremely important in encouraging new research in every kind of MD, increasing awareness of the disease among policy-makers, and providing resources to positively impact the everyday life of patients living with MD. This can be a rewarding area for patients who wish to be involved in changing their own lives and those of others afflicted by this group of diseases.

## Non-U.S. Patient Advocacy Groups

Because some of the forms of MD are so rare, little information is available in the U.S.; therefore, a patient with a very rare form of MD may need to look outside of the U.S. to get additional information. Although beyond the scope of this chapter to discuss in detail, one Website worth mentioning is Treat-NMD. Treat-NMD (www. treat-nmd.eu) is a neuromuscular network that provides a list of global registries that can be accessed at http://www.treat-nmd.eu/resources/patient-registries/list/. Queries can be made by going to the disease information tab, picking a disease, and then on left-hand side menu, a "patient organizations" tab can be clicked to view the worldwide list of organizations for that disease.

---

**Learning About FSHD: Tips for Patients**

*Meredith L. Huml*

As a MD sufferer—I was diagnosed with FSHD at Duke University's MDA Center in 2003—the best advice I could offer someone who is newly diagnosed would be, "Don't hesitate to educate yourself on your disease." Figuring out what exactly you are dealing with and how you can help yourself and your loved ones will make the situation easier to cope with as a whole.

*Connect with Advocacy Groups & Other Patients*
Fortunately, awareness of MD continues to grow. Scientists continue to produce more findings and hopefully one day, there will be a cure for every type

(continued)

(continued)
of MD. As our world becomes more connected, it is easier to read up on updates in research, learn the symptoms and causes of your malady, and connect with others through social media. Patient advocacy is vital in fighting MD, as it is with any medical condition, especially those with limited awareness and no cure at this point in time. There is always the option of making a donation to organizations that fight against MD, setting up a fundraiser for the cause, or working at a summer camp for children afflicted. Using your voice is an important tool as well. The MDA provides a page in which you can find your elected officials who vote on important pieces of legislation affecting MD patients and their families.

*Ask for Help When You Need It*
As a patient, I understand that this disease comes with more than just physical side effects. It can be humiliating, frightening, stressful, disheartening, and confusing. I was diagnosed with depression in high school after I began to accept the changes going on in my body, and when I began to try and accept and recognize my limitations. Even without the daily struggle of coping with MD, it can sometimes be difficult and embarrassing to admit our weaknesses and to ask for help when we need it. We want to be independent, we want to take care of things ourselves, we want to say "I did this for myself. I didn't need help."

I am still learning how to ask for help. I am learning how to undermine my stubbornness, I am learning to talk about and admit openly the simple truth that I am physically weaker than most people that I encounter. I am learning to offer a compromise when invited to do things I may not have the strength to do, or learn how to tell others I'm going to have to "sit this one out," I am learning to watch others run and dance and climb with joy instead of resentment, jealousy, and anger.

*Try Exploring New Pastimes*
It is easy to feel cheated when you don't have the same opportunities and it is easy to feel excluded. I began dance when I was three years old. I fell in love with it. It was a way to be active in a fashion that I felt coincided with my very soul, and it was a way for me to get stress out. I took tap dance classes, I took ballet, I took hip-hop, modern/contemporary. Being in a studio was like being at a different kind of home. When I was forced to take a lower level dance class as a sophomore in high school, the same one I had taken as a freshman, I was angry. I couldn't physically keep up with the higher level classes, and it tore at me. I had been a dancer for years and years, I could choreograph a routine in a short amount of time, I knew how to do all the moves, I heard counts and beats in every song I heard. I day-dreamed routines in my mind, I couldn't listen to a song without wanting to move some part of me.

(continued)

(continued)

After my sophomore year, I admitted defeat to myself. I stopped dance altogether. I canceled my subscription to my dance magazine and shoved my tights and leotards in the bottom of my drawer. To give up something that seems like your life, something that you're passionate about, is torturous. It brings about some of the emotions I previously mentioned. As someone with MD, you are most likely able to relate. To give up something like that, and on top of that, sometimes even simple daily tasks, is a complete life changer. And seeing others accomplish things you wish to as well is frustrating.

*Enjoy Simple Pleasures*

There is, however, good news. There is always a silver lining if you choose to look close enough. You did not choose this, your loved ones who suffer from MD did not chose this. Blaming yourself, blaming others, and being angry is something that will cripple you even more. Let any anger you feel serve as motivation for something great, or throw it away. You may be unable to run down the soccer field, you may not be able to climb mountains by yourself, you may have to give up things you find hard to. There are other things you can try, other hobbies you can find. I threw myself into art and writing, and found that I have somewhat of a talent for both that I am working on furthering developing. Negative emotions are hurtful, but you can put them into words that others may relate to, you can let them flow through a paintbrush, you can sing them for a loved one. There is still a beautiful life that you can fit into just as easily as anyone else, and you are no lower than anyone else just because maybe you need help reaching for that cup on the top shelf. You have a unique perspective as a person with MD. You may possess a greater appreciation of the simpler things in life, you may be less judgmental as you understand that everyone has their own struggles in life, and just because you can't always see or understand them does not mean they do not exist. You may be more compassionate due to the fact the compassion towards yourself is greatly appreciated, that when someone asks for help it might mean the world to them just as my friends piggy-backing me up hills without annoyance or frustration means the world to me. You may learn how to cope better, or you may develop better coping skills from having to deal with so much yourself on a daily basis.

I struggled many years worried about what I later discovered were rather silly things. People who truly love you DO want to help you, even if they don't always know the right way, the right things to say or do. While I was generally embarrassed and felt sometimes annoying, I've been told many times things like "It's not even a big deal. It's cute anyway! I'd give you piggy-back rides regardless if you wanted."

It takes courage to be open. Walking in public places might get you many stares or whispers. I've heard countless mentions of how thin I am, or how my

(continued)

(continued)

gait is slightly off. While it is sometimes hurtful, I've learned to either address the situation by using it as an opportunity to politely educate someone, or simply ignore it. What others say of you says more about them than it does you. Some people simply haven't heard of MD. It doesn't necessarily mean they are uncaring or cruel. A girl I once sat by in a class of mine used to tell me nearly every day that I should eat more, because I looked sickly. For several weeks I either laughed it off or mumbled back things like "yeah, maybe." After a while I finally mustered the courage to tell her that I was only thin because of my condition, and I actually ate more than a man going through college. Not only did she feel extremely guilty (which wasn't my goal), but she learned something new and started helping me gather my things after class, offering to carry my books if I needed.

*Smile the Best Way You Can*
Never take situations like this personally; you are beautiful no matter your capabilities or your appearance. Living with any disease is hard. MD has posed many obstacles for me, has brought many tears, and has made me question things I probably normally wouldn't without it. I am growing a greater appreciation for MD every day, however odd that may sound. It has taught me compassion, it has taught me forgiveness, it has taught me humility, courage, and appreciation. Life does not often go as planned, and we must learn to accept that and use it to our advantage. So, while people telling to smile bigger has always bugged me due to the fact I've lost some muscles in my cheeks, I urge you to smile in the best way you can. It is okay to hurt, it is okay to cry, it is okay to feel sad and lazy some days. It will rain some days, just remember the good weather, and know that it is coming. Don't be afraid to let others help you, and don't be afraid to offer your help to others. I wish you much peace, plenty of love, and safety in your journey.

# Chapter 14
# Global and National Patient Registries

Raymond A. Huml

## Introduction

An muscular dystrophy (MD) patient registry is a collection of secondary data related to patients (and therefore may include family members) with one of the nine types of MD. Registries can vary in sophistication from simple MS Excel spreadsheets that can be accessed only by a small group of physicians, to very complex databases that are accessed online across multiple institutions.

Due to the small numbers of patients with MD, it is important to identify patients quickly in order to share rapidly evolving scientific advances with them, advocate for them, and provide opportunities to advance our scientific knowledge about each type of MD so that, ultimately, a cure can be found.

Registries can play multiple roles including identifying MD patients for scientific research, clinical trials, and later, as products/drugs are approved for the treatment of MD, in the post-marketing surveillance of pharmaceuticals. Registries can also provide healthcare providers or patients with reminders of the need to undergo certain tests in order to reach quality goals.

Registries are less complex and simpler to set up than an electronic medical record, which keeps track of all the patients a doctor follows, while a registry only keeps track of a small subpopulation of patients with a specific condition.

Currently, many registries are only offered in one geographic area or for just one or two types of MD. The Muscular Dystrophy Association (MDA), the largest MD patient advocacy group in the world, recognizing how difficult it is to identify and find patients to study treatments for MD, is attempting to remedy this disparity and has posted two important news items applicable to patients afflicted with MD [1]:

R.A. Huml, M.S., D.V.M., R.A.C. (✉)
Biosimilars Center of Excellence, Quintiles Inc., 4820 Emperor Boulevard,
Durham, NC 27703, USA
e-mail: raymond.huml@quintiles.com

© Springer International Publishing Switzerland 2015
R.A. Huml (ed.), *Muscular Dystrophy*, DOI 10.1007/978-3-319-17362-7_14

1. The first, and most recent news item, is the solicitation for a patient registry and world map of people with certain types of myopathies (e.g., centronuclear [CNM]/myotubular myopathy [MTM]), which are being developed and are seeking participation from people with these disorders or their family members. This database is designed to allow researchers to better understand certain diseases and locate participants for clinical trials and other research studies.

   • The registry site will initially make possible the study of the natural history of each disease, which is the first step towards understanding the progression or course of the disease. This is especially important when determining if a new treatment or therapy has the potential to alter or stop disease progression (as compared with using a placebo or sugar pill) in a clinical study. Natural history is defined by the National Cancer Institute [2] as "a study that follows a group of people over time who have, or are at risk of developing, a specific medical condition or disease. A study that collects health information to understand how the medical condition or disease develops and how to treat it." An alternative is the definition provided by Posada and Groft [3]: "The natural course of a disease from the time immediately prior to its inception, progressing through its presymptomatic phase and different clinical stages to the point where it has ended and the patient is either cured, chronically disabled or dead without external intervention."
   • Given the potential for this information to be misused (e.g., individuals being targeted by insurance companies), patient privacy is protected and de-identified information will be shared only with "selected members of the research community" and a Scientific Advisory Board.
   • Registrants will receive email updates on research progress and be notified of trial participation opportunities. A de-identified "pin" will be added to the global map after a participant has given his or her approval for the posting.
   • "This information is crucial for helping us to understand the demographics of our community," says the foundation's website. "If you know of anyone affected with CNM/MTM, please direct them to this website and ask them to register."

2. Currently, the lack of a fully operational central registry database for patients with MD is problematic. With so many smaller registries scattered across the U.S., it is difficult for researchers to find enough patients to fulfill enrollment requirements for a proposed MD clinical study. Therefore, to address this issue, Quintiles, a biopharmaceutical services company, and the MDA announced a new partnership in October 2013 [4], to develop and implement the U.S. Neuromuscular Disease Registry, a patient registry that will play an important role in determining effective treatments for people with MD and related muscle diseases.

   • According to MDA's Website, "We are making remarkable progress in researching new lifesaving treatments and cures for neuromuscular diseases as we move from bench to bedside in clinical trials," said MDA Executive Vice President & Chief Medical and Scientific Officer Valerie Cwik, M.D. "We are committed to changing and saving the lives of the individuals and families we serve, and the U.S. Neuromuscular Disease Registry brings us one step closer to answering critical clinical and research questions that will improve quality of care."

- Quintiles was awarded the project based on its depth of experience in post-marketing research, multistakeholder strategy, and systems-oriented approach to registry design and development [3]. "Patient registries are an increasingly important component of real-world evidence development for understanding the cause of disease and identifying effective treatments," said Richard Gliklich, M.D., then president of Quintiles Real World & Late Phase Research. "In designing the U.S. Neuromuscular Disease Registry, our goal is to create a research and collaboration platform that will enable physicians, patients, caregivers and others involved in MDA's mission to collaborate to advance new treatments for patients."
- MDA will use the registry to study the natural history of MD and related muscle diseases, collect information on practice patterns, inform care guidelines, and improve quality of care for patients. The registry is currently available at 25 medical clinics within the organization's national network, with plans to expand to their full network of 200 clinics. It will gather data in a common format across neuromuscular diseases, starting with amyotrophic lateral sclerosis (ALS), Becker muscular dystrophy/Duchene muscular dystrophy (BMD/DMD), and spinal muscular atrophy (SMA), with plans to collect data on three other neuromuscular diseases within three years.

Other registries are available throughout the world and may be specific for certain types of MD [5–7]. These registries can help patients with MD network with others who have the same disease or have a special interest in developing therapies for patients afflicted with a certain type of MD (e.g., caregivers, physicians, and research scientists).

Take, for example, The Myotubular and Centronuclear Myopathy Patient Registry (also referred to as "MTM and CNM Registry"), which is an international database managed from the UK and operated by the Myotubular Trust. According to their Website, the registry was developed in partnership with TREAT-NMD (Neuro Muscular Network) and with a number of leading neuromuscular researchers and plans to:

- Help identify patients for relevant clinical trials as they become available
- Encourage further research into MTM and CNM
- Provide researchers with specific patient information to support their research
- Assist doctors and other health professionals by providing them with up-to-date information on managing MTM and CNM, to help them deliver better standards of care for their patients.

- The requirements for registration include:

  - All patients, with a MTM or CNM diagnosis, which has been confirmed via genetic testing or muscle biopsy.
  - Any carrier females of x-linked MTM, especially if they have manifested MTM type symptoms.
  - Any patient who is deceased, but who had a confirmed diagnosis.
  - Any patient who wishes to receive information only.

- Their aim is, in part, to "get a good insight into the numbers of people affected."

Another example is a patient registry for myotonic dystrophy (DM) and FSHD which was started in the U.S. as part of a National Institutes of Health (NIH) grant (e.g., NIH contract # N01-AR-02250). Starting in 2001, the project established a national research registry for people with the diseases and their families. The registry—established by the National Institute of Arthritis and Musculoskeletal and Skin Diseases (NIAMS) and the National Institute of Neurological Disorders and Stroke (NINDS), both parts of the NIH—is based at the University of Rochester (Rochester, NY).

Registry scientists sought out and classified patients with clinically diagnosed forms of myotonic dystrophy (DM) and FSHD and stored their medical and family history data. The registry is a central information source where researchers can obtain data for analysis associated with these diseases.

The registry's scientific advisory committee made recommendations about enrollment criteria, monitored and improved ways to recruit patients and investigators, and assessed progress. It also revised and extended methods for collecting and handling data and determined possible clinical studies.

NIAMS Director Stephen I. Katz, M.D., Ph.D., said, "This national registry will be an important resource to provide hope to families and encourage scientists in finding a cure for these two disabling diseases. It will also hasten the course of research for more in-depth answers to what happens in muscular dystrophy."

Richard Moxley III, M.D., was the lead investigator for the registry. "Research has uncovered recent clues to genetic, chromosomal and DNA errors in those with DM and FSHD," he said. "I am pleased to lead scientists in collecting and analyzing new research data for better treatments for these two diseases."

DM and FSHD are two of the nine types of MD. They can be detected through testing at birth and may be passed from one generation to the next. Both cause progressive, disabling weakness. In addition, DM sometimes results in sudden death.

Similar to the MDA in the U.S., the EU has important groups dedicated to helping those afflicted with MD, such as Treat-NMD. This group's Web site posts its mission statement as follows:

> TREAT-NMD is a network for the neuromuscular field that provides an infrastructure to ensure that the most promising new therapies reach patients as quickly as possible. Since its launch in January 2007 the network's focus has been on the development of tools that industry, clinicians and scientists need to bring novel therapeutic approaches through preclinical development and into the clinic, and on establishing best-practice care for neuromuscular patients worldwide.

The Web site also includes a useful section on patient registries that demonstrates the fundamental thinking—and potential scientific utility—of any registry:

- A patient registry collects information about patients who are affected by a particular condition.
- When planning a clinical trial, it is very important that eligible patients can be found and contacted quickly. The best way for this to happen is through a database or "registry" that contains all the information that researchers will need. Patients' clinical and genetic details are collected and made easily available for the researchers.
- Scientific advances over recent years have led to substantial changes in the treatment of many neuromuscular diseases. Several new therapeutic strategies which target specific genetic defects are being developed. For some of these treatments, plans are already in place for large studies involving patients from more than one country.
- Any potential new treatment needs to be tested under strictly controlled circumstances to make sure that not only are participants safe but, that any notable changes can be attributed to the treatment and not to external factors. This allows researchers to ensure that all potential new therapies are both safe and effective.
- Due to the nature of rare diseases, scientific approaches differ from those used for common diseases. Finding enough patients who might be eligible to participate in trials for rare neuromuscular conditions can take years without a patient registry, delaying the testing of potential therapies.

Because there are multiple registries, it can be confusing for both the newly diagnosed patient and the caregiver. In general, for those who are unfamiliar with a certain type of MD, most patient advocacy groups provide links and post information for patients and their caregivers [8]. For example, the FSH Society Website has a "For Patients" link that lists how FSHD researchers and clinical trials are connected through their own list as well as their connection to the NIH. According to their Website:

- A disease registry or patient registry is a database of information on patients with a particular disease, such as FSHD, that can be accessed and used by researchers, clinicians, and physicians interested in working on the disease. Registries are especially valuable in diseases like FSHD where access to patients and materials is limited. The collected information contained within the registry is used to increase the understanding of FSHD by allowing doctors, clinicians, and researchers to access patients and biomaterials. Many more research projects and avenues of investigation will result from FSHD patients and their families signing up and becoming involved!
- There are several disease research or patient registries available for FSHD in the U.S.:
  - The FSH Society maintains a FSHD registry of patients and families wishing to become involved in research.

– The NIH funds the National Registry of Myotonic Dystrophy and Facioscapulohumeral Muscular Dystrophy Patients and Family Members. The National Registry helps individuals and families with FSHD participate in research on their disease. It helps investigators accomplish their research by connecting them with people who have FSHD and it acts as a resource to facilitate more research on FSHD.

## Summary

Due to the small numbers of patients with MD, it is important for patients with MD (and their caregivers) to be aware of patient and disease registries in order to access the latest scientific information and be provided with the opportunity to become part of scientific investigations. Registries can be a good way to gain access to clinical studies which, after a positive risk/benefit assessment is made by the patient and the patient's caregivers, provide opportunities to obtain disease modifying, or possibly even curative, therapies.

For patients living in the U.S., contacting the MDA is the logical first step to find a registry for a particular type of MD. Other smaller patient advocacy groups, such as the FSH Society, may offer more patient-specific details, as they are sometimes staffed or founded by individuals afflicted by the disease.

## References

1. MDA, Quest. http://quest.mda.org/news/cnm-mtm-registry-world-map-seek-participants. Accessed 9 Nov 2014.
2. National Cancer Institute, August 2014.
3. Posada de la Paz M, Groft SC, editors. Rare diseases epidemiology, Vol. 6862010, XXII, 542; 2010.
4. Quintiles selected by Muscular Dystrophy Association to develop US Disease Registry. [news release]. Quintiles Media Relations. 8 Oct 2013. http://www.quintiles.com/library/press-releases/quintiles-selected-by-muscular-dystrophy-association-to-develop-u-s-disease-registry/. Accessed 25 Oct 2013.
5. The Myotubular and Centronuclear Myopathy Registry. http://www.mtmcnmregistry.org/. Accessed 22 Nov 2013.
6. National Registry Established for Two Muscular Dystrophy Types [news release]. National Institute of Arthritis and Musculoskeletal and Skin Diseases Office of Communications. 11 Dec 2000. http://www.niams.nih.gov/News_and_Events/Press_Releases/2000/12_11.asp. Accessed 22 Nov 2013.
7. Muscular Dystrophy Campaign Registry (UK). http://www.treat-nmd.eu/. Accessed 22 Nov 2013.
8. FSH Society. For patients. http://www.fshsociety.org/pages/patPatReg.html. Accessed 10 Nov 2014.

# Chapter 15
# Summary

Raymond A. Huml

Muscular dystrophy (MD) comprises a group of diseases that are clinically manifested as progressive muscle weakness with associated loss of mobility, agility, and body movements due to defects in genes for the production of muscle proteins. Devastating to patients, families, and caregivers, and clinically known for over 150 years, there is as yet no cure for MD.

Despite the challenges to finding a cure, however, the proteins and structures involved in certain disease processes are increasingly being elucidated, raising the number of potential pharmaceutical targets, and resulting in heightened interest in investment, partnership, and collaboration. In addition, several companies pursing potential treatments for MD have advanced to the Phase II and III stages of clinical drug development, and one product may be fully approved in the near future.

There are at least nine major types of MD: Duchenne (DMD), Becker (BMD), congenital, distal, Emery-Dreifuss, facioscapulohumeral (FSHD or FSH), limb-girdle, myotonic dystrophy, and oculopharyngeal. Most of the pharmaceutical and regulatory efforts to date have focused on DMD, because it is the most severe and because of considerable scientific advances regarding its pathology, and BMD, because its disease mechanism is related to DMD.

MD can be inherited in three ways: (1) autosomal inheritance (from a normal gene from one parent and an abnormal gene from another parent), (2) autosomal recessive inheritance (both parents carry and pass on the faulty gene), and (3) X-linked recessive inheritance (when a mother carries the affected gene and passes it on to her son). Sporadic cases may also arise as a result of de novo mutation, in the absence of any family history of affected individuals. The distribution of weakness in MDs includes a limb-girdle pattern, with shoulder and hip girdle muscle

R.A. Huml, M.S., D.V.M., R.A.C. (✉)
Biosimilars Center of Excellence, Quintiles Inc., 4820 Emperor Boulevard,
Durham, NC 27703, USA
e-mail: raymond.huml@quintiles.com

© Springer International Publishing Switzerland 2015
R.A. Huml (ed.), *Muscular Dystrophy*, DOI 10.1007/978-3-319-17362-7_15

involvement; a humeroperoneal pattern, with predominantly triceps, biceps, and peroneal muscles weakness; or a distal pattern, with distal weakness in the legs and arms. The prevalence of MD ranges from 1.3 to 96.2 per million, with DMD being most prevalent among boys during childhood, and myotonic dystrophy as one of the more common forms of MDs worldwide. Traditionally, the classification of MD is based on a combination of clinical and pathological criteria, including age of onset and distribution of muscle weakness, the extent of disease progression, associated symptoms, systemic features, family history, serum creatine kinase, muscle histology, as well as electromyography and nerve conduction studies (EMG/NCS). Increasingly, diagnosis requires genetic confirmation, as there can be considerable variations and overlaps in the clinical phenotypes.

FSHD is a complex, inheritable muscle disease. Although frequently cited as the third most common type of MD in older reports, many newer sources rank FSHD as the most prevalent type of MD, occurring at a rate of some 7 cases/1,000 persons, as compared with DMD/BMD (5 cases/1,000) and myotonic dystrophy (4.5 cases/1,000). The identification of FSHD as the most common type of MD has important ramifications, for example, when allocating future Federal (U.S.) funding for research, and in terms of the potential market size for future FSHD treatments. FSHD has only recently attracted attention from the pharmaceutical industry, largely due to significant advances in the understanding of the gene/mechanism of disease, including over-expression of a protein called DUX4. Most individuals with FSHD inherit the mutation from a parent with the disease, with 10–33% of all FSHD cases resulting from a de novo (or sporadic) mutation. The major symptom of FSHD is progressive weakening and loss of skeletal muscles. The usual location of these weaknesses at onset is the origin of the name: face (facio), shoulder girdle (scapulo), and upper arms (humeral). There is currently no disease modifying treatment or cure for FSHD. Most treatments proposed to "treat" FSHD have not yet been tested in randomized clinical trials. These may include: hormone supplementation, protein supplements (creatinine monohydrate), or drugs used to decrease inflammation (e.g., prednisone). To better understand and validate their use, many are now being properly investigated in clinical trials.

Duchenne and Becker MD are allelic disorders caused by mutations of the DMD gene located on Xp21, which encodes for the dystrophin protein. DMD is the most common form of MD in childhood, with an estimated incidence of 1 per 3,500 live-born males, and a pooled prevalence of DMD of 4.78 per 100,000 males worldwide. BMD is a generally milder and more variable form of dystrophinopathy, with an incidence of 1 in 18,518 male births, and a pooled prevalence of 1.53 per 100,000 males worldwide. Diagnosis is based on careful review of the clinical features and confirmed by additional investigations including muscle biopsy and/ or genetic testing. Suspicion of the diagnosis of DMD is usually triggered in one of three ways, including (1) most commonly, the observation of abnormal muscle function with signs of proximal muscle weakness in a male child; (2) the detection of elevated serum creatine kinase as part of routine screening; or (3) the presence of elevated liver enzymes including aspartate aminotransferase and alanine aminotransferase. Current strategies include promoting proper nutrition, delaying onset of complications, and optimizing health outcomes through on-going support. Pharmaceutical interventions include corticosteroids for skeletal muscle weakness and afterload reduction for cardiomyopathy. Early recognition and precise genetic diagnosis may allow for new therapeutic options for DMD.

Even though there is currently no cure, respiratory intervention and other supportive strategies have led to improved survival and better health-related quality of life for many affected individuals. For example, patients with DMD lived on average until their late teens in the 1950s; today, they typically live until their late 20s or 30s, which is largely attributable to better supportive care. This may include noninvasive ventilation during the day, and at night, orthopedic care and preventive measures. Current treatment is focused on symptomatic management and rehabilitation, and monitoring for disease complications.

Accurate diagnosis is important as a first step for managing MD. This involves a targeted history and examination, biochemical and genetic testing—sometimes with additional testing such as muscle biopsy—neurophysiological assessment, and muscle imaging. Muscle biopsy used to be the gold standard; however, it is increasingly being replaced by genetic testing. Muscle imaging is becoming more widely accepted as it is noninvasive and various forms of MD often result in unique patterns.

There has been progress in ICH countries toward issuing regulatory guidance for development of drugs for certain types of MD. The EU is most advanced, with draft guidance for DMD and BMD issued in 2013, and a concept paper published in 2011. The U.S. seems to be taking a conservative approach, relying on current programs—such as Fast Track Designation, Breakthrough Therapy Designation, Accelerated Approval, and Priority Review—to help sponsors of MD therapies gain U.S. registration. In an unprecedented move, the FDA solicited the first-ever draft guidance for industry written on behalf of a patient advocacy group with a focus on DMD, although it is possible that the Agency may choose not to formally adopt the proposed guidance. Since there is no other official guidance in the U.S., the PPMD document serves as a precedent for other types of MDs. As of April 2015, there are no disease-modifying products approved for the treatment of MD, but that situation may soon change. In May 2014, reversing an earlier rejection, the EU Committee for Medicinal Products for Human Use (CHMP) recommended early (conditional) approval for PTC Therapeutics' ataluren, a potential treatment for DMD. If the European Commission supports this decision, ataluren would be the first product approved, albeit conditionally, for MD—until the final Phase III data is available.

No MD products have yet been approved in the U.S., and significant hurdles remain to gaining regulatory approval of products to treat all patients with MD. A major challenge in developing therapies is the considerable variation in the severity and rate of disease progression between individuals. Other hurdles include: difficulty in defining and measuring the rate of change in this slowly progressing disease; variation in the goals of treatment at each stage of MD; the lack of protein identification and complete understanding of the mechanism of action in certain types of MD (e.g., FSHD); lack of regulatory agreement on primary and secondary endpoints in the U.S.; and the fact that few patients are available or eligible for study in clinical trials. Once drug developers identify enough patients to study, but before moving to clinical trials, they need to have a minimum understanding of the natural history for each type of MD and make sure that the preclinical data package justifies the risk/benefit for patients (and caregivers). Until clinical endpoints and other key clinical trial design features are provided in U.S. and EU regulatory guidance, sponsors of drugs will need to collaborate with regulatory agencies on a case-by-case basis and early solicitation is encouraged. Despite the challenges, substantial progress has been made and there are a number of late stage candidates in clinical development primarily for DMD. More work is urgently needed to address the other eight types of MD.

Regarding patient advocacy groups, the first point of call for information and support for newly-diagnosed MD patients and their caregivers in the U.S., is the Muscular Dystrophy Association (MDA, www.mda.org). Other disease-specific groups for several of the nine forms of MD are presented in Chapter 13.

MD registries—collections of secondary data related to patients with one of the nine types of MD—can vary in sophistication from simple spreadsheets accessible only by a small group of physicians, to complex databases accessed online across multiple institutions. Registries can help identify MD patients for scientific research, clinical trials, and later, as products/drugs are approved for the treatment of MD, in the post-marketing surveillance of pharmaceuticals. Registries can also give healthcare providers or patients reminders of the need to undergo certain tests in order to reach quality goals. At present, many registries cover only one geographic area or one or two types of MD. The MDA is attempting to remedy this disparity with two initiatives. First, it is seeking participation from patients with certain myopathies in a patient registry and world map. This database is designed to allow researchers to better understand certain diseases and locate participants for clinical trials and other research studies. Second, to address the lack of a fully operational central registry database for patients with MD, the MDA and Quintiles, a biopharmaceutical services company, formed a partnership in October 2013 to develop and implement the U.S. Neuromuscular Disease Registry.

At no time in the history of MD has the future looked brighter. With over 240 studies listed in the U.S.—and at least 11 candidates in the later phases of drug development (e.g., Phase II or Phase III)—the stage is set for positive change. More groundwork is needed, however, such as the conduct of natural history studies, establishment of more global patient registries, and completion of additional genetic and molecular studies, to better understand MD and to identify promising targets. Indeed, it has historically proven difficult to find preclinical and animal models of disease. Several promising approaches to DMD are in the pipeline, including: "exon skipping" drug candidates, which target the mutation that occurs in the gene for dystrophin in individuals with DMD; gene therapy, aimed at introducing a healthy synthetic copy of the dystrophin gene into the muscles to restore production of dystrophin; "reading through stop signals" by targeting a specific type of mistake in the genetic code called a nonsense mutation, which prevents the production of full-length functional proteins; stem cell therapy, where donor cells are injected with the aim of creating healthy muscle fibers; utrophin upregulation, aimed at increasing levels of utrophin, a protein that is functionally similar to dystrophin; and reducing muscle damage. As ongoing studies are completed, it is hoped that the mechanism of disease will become better elucidated, more targets will be identified, and more companies will be willing to invest in clinical trials.

# Index

© Springer International Publishing Switzerland 2015
R.A. Huml (ed.), *Muscular Dystrophy*, DOI 10.1007/978-3-319-17362-7

Printed by Printforce, the Netherlands